OPEN HEART WARRIOR SPIRIT

A MAN'S GUIDE TO LIVING WITH CANCER

#KFG

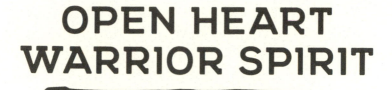

TREVOR MAXWELL

MAN UP TO CANCER
MANUPTOCANCER.COM

Published in the United States by
Man Up to Cancer
manuptocancer.com

Managed and edited by Danielle Derbenti
Copyedited by Janelle Bretz
Book design by Trese Gloriod
Cover design by Kelin Welborn

ISBN: 979-8-9871780-0-3

DEDICATION

To Sarah, Sage, and Elsie.
Thank you for being my people.

TABLE OF CONTENTS

PREFACE

FOR MEN FACING CANCER, there's an old road to travel.

On that road, men walk alone. We are told to toughen up. Don't burden others. Handle the situation. Don't talk about it.

Sounds like the hero in an old-fashioned Western movie, right?

The trouble is, when it comes to cancer, that old road often leads to tragic endings. Men who isolate during cancer are more likely to experience anxiety, depression, broken relationships, and emotional turmoil every step of the way. They are also more likely to die sooner, compared to men who are not isolated.

I'm inviting you to consider a new road.

On the new road for men impacted by cancer, we share the burden with others, including men who are going through the same challenges. We engage with communities and resources that give us our best chance at survival. We acknowledge the physical and emotional pain we're going through, and we use tools to cope.

We don't walk this road alone.

By sharing my experiences as a cancer patient, I hope you'll gain insights into what many guys go through, as well as practical strategies to improve your lives.

In March of 2018, I was diagnosed with colon cancer, which ultimately spread to my liver and throughout my abdomen. As of this writing, in the fall of 2022, I have been through five major surgeries, one clinical trial, and more than 50 rounds of chemotherapy and immunotherapy. Nearly five years have passed, and I have not had a break from my quest to be cancer-free.

In January of 2020, I launched Man Up to Cancer, a support community emboldened by the tagline Open Heart, Warrior Spirit.

What started as a small gathering of a few guys with cancer, Man Up to Cancer has grown steadily over the past few years, mostly through word of mouth. Our members connect on social media and in person through local meet-ups and an annual retreat.

The core of it all is the Howling Place. This is so much more than another Facebook group. It's a place of brotherhood and growth for male cancer patients, survivors, and caregivers from around the world.

The resources we provide are also growing. We launched our Chemo Backpack program in 2022, sending backpacks filled with comfort items and practical gifts to men going through chemotherapy. We've been fortunate to partner with some of the most influential companies and organizations in cancer care.

—————————————

There's a wolf on the cover of this book.

If one wolf is sick or injured, others guard him and encourage him toward health. If the wolf dies, others are there to provide kinship. The pack does not abandon a member.

When life gets hard, we all need our wolfpacks.

We need our packmates to share the path with us, to play and wonder and mourn. We need them to make this human experience worth the pain that a cancer diagnosis and treatment bring. Man Up to Cancer has given us our pack.

—————————————

Before you decide to read further, you should know a bit more about me.

I've worked as a telephone operator; on a construction crew; and as a communications director, freelance writer, and PR consultant. I was a newspaper journalist for nearly 15 years. I married my high school sweetheart and we have two teenage daughters. We live on the coast of Maine.

I love splitting wood with axes and mauls. I have a tattoo on my shoulder of my ancestral castle, a lion, and a warrior's shield. I have a tattoo of a wolf on my forearm. One of my favorite jobs was working on a house-framing construction crew with my uncle. I'm 6'4", 230 pounds, and I will wrestle if necessary.

Also, I love English literature, the Indigo Girls, and *The Notebook*. When I was seven, my two favorite activities were baseball and playing Barbie with my cousins. When I used to watch *Little Bear* with my daughters, I'm pretty sure I enjoyed it more than they did. I can't read *The Giving Tree* without weeping.

Is there room for all of this under your mental tent? Can men—even those of us going through cancer—retain our rough-and-tough edges while also opening our hearts to one another, without shame?

If you believe yes, then by all means read on. If no, then maybe this isn't the book for you.

Or maybe it is, and you just don't know it yet....

Trevor Maxwell
Cape Elizabeth, Maine
October, 2022

CHAPTER 1

MAN OF THE LIVING ROOM FLOOR

IMAGINE A RUGGED, 6'4", 230-pound man, crumpled on his living room floor.

Sobbing uncontrollably. Clutching t-shirts belonging to his wife and young daughters. On his knees, rocking back and forth, unable to function. Full of shame and self-loathing.

> *I just want to disappear into the woods and never come back.*
>
> *I don't want to be a burden to my wife and kids anymore.*
>
> *Cancer is going to kill me, and I'm going to leave them all alone.*
>
> *I'm a failure.*

Those are the words on repeat in his mind—the full expression of animal grief, so deep and so bottomless that he can't imagine there will ever be a way out. He barely eats. He can't make a phone call, send a text, or leave the house.

That was me in September of 2018, six months into my diagnosis of stage IV colon cancer.

I was 41 years old, a husband and father raising a family at our home on the coast of Maine. I had gone through the shock of diagnosis, a surgery to remove more than a foot of my large intestine, and the relentless nausea of chemotherapy. At that point I was getting ready for another surgery to remove tumors from my liver.

Entire days would pass this way, in heartbreak, tears, and silence. My wife, Sarah, an elementary school teacher, and our daughters, then 13 and 11, would get up early and head out for their schools. I would stay in bed and pull the covers over my head, pretending I didn't hear the bustle downstairs.

Then I'd sit outside in a camp chair, staring blankly at the first leaves that had fallen in the yard, consumed for hours by thoughts of despair.

My mind would drift into the past, to our lives before cancer, as if somehow there was a way back.

I felt that getting cancer in the prime of my life had somehow been my fault. And now, here I was, failing at coping with my diagnosis—"checking out"—and pushing away my family, my friends, and my whole life prior to cancer.

I would try to engage in activities that once meant something to me, like watching a Red Sox game, eating a favorite food, taking a nature walk, or simply hanging out with friends. But I wasn't really there: It was a dream, and I was trapped inside a glass jar, still able to see the world moving around me, but unable to participate.

I thought to myself, "I don't know how others do this, but I'm sure this is not how a man is supposed to respond to cancer."

What I didn't know at the time was that my grief was a common response for the newly diagnosed, especially for those of us with young children who face cancer at a relatively young age.

I didn't know then that men facing cancer tend to struggle with a loss of identity and have higher rates of mental health problems than women facing cancer. There are thousands, if not millions, of men who are emotionally crushed by the diagnosis of a life-threatening illness. At the time, I just thought I was weak.

I didn't know any of this because, well, most guys just don't let you see their pain. And they certainly don't share about it publicly.

We get the diagnosis, retreat into our man caves—and many of us never make it back out.

THE DIAGNOSIS

Exhaustion was my only symptom before my cancer diagnosis.

Prior to 2017, I always had plenty of energy. I had been a three-sport athlete in high school and played club sports in college. I was a physical person by nature.

Like many families in Maine, we heat with wood. It was never a problem for me to use the chainsaw and wood splitter for hours at a time. Manual labor was a joy, and I even spent a few years working on my uncle's house-framing crew, lugging plywood and firing nail guns. At home I would swim and bike and play with our daughters, Sage and Elsie.

Over the course of 2017, though, I felt the fatigue creeping in.

When I carried boxes full of wood from the barn to the house, I would stop more often to catch my breath. In the middle of the day, I would have to lie down for a nap. I didn't tell anyone how I was feeling. I felt guilty that I wasn't being productive enough.

I figured I was tired because, you know, life. I was hitting my 40s, with a wife and two young kids, and was running my own business as a writer and public relations consultant. I was also no stranger to chronic, low-level anxiety, which I had experienced most of my adult life. So as the fatigue intensified, I chalked it up to age and mental health. I thought I was just in an extended funk.

But my body wasn't recovering from breaks. By the early months of 2018, my resting heart rate had jumped from around 50 to around 70. I'd climb one flight of stairs and spend two minutes with my hands on my knees.

4

After months of tough-guy stubbornness, in March of 2018 I finally called my primary care physician, Dr. Tara Pelletier. Tara was our family's doctor and also a family friend.

"You're probably fine," Tara told me. "But let's get blood work done to see if there are any red flags." On a Wednesday, I went for my blood draw.

That Friday, Sarah and I took Sage and Elsie out of school and went to a local ski mountain for a day of skiing. We had been feeling that we needed a family break to have some fun. I was exhausted, just like every day back then, but I bulled through, even when it felt like my heart was pounding out of my chest.

Tara called that afternoon and left a message. I didn't see the notification until we were just about home, late on Friday evening.

"Give me a call when you get this message. It doesn't matter what time it is," she said. "We need to talk about your lab results."

I thought, "Well, that's probably not good."

I waited for Sarah and the girls to get inside. Then I called. Tara told me there was hardly any iron in my blood; I was extremely anemic. I was not in urgent need of a blood transfusion, she said, but I was close. All of my fatigue, she said, was being caused by the anemia.

"Have you noticed any bleeding recently?" she asked.

I hadn't.

"These numbers tell me you must be losing blood some-where. Possibly your digestive tract. I'm going to schedule you for a colonoscopy ASAP. Don't do anything strenuous."

Damn.

When I got off the call, I stood outside for a long time, lis-tening to the muffled sounds of the girls in the house getting ready for bed. I watched my breath in the cold air, rising slowly toward the stars.

"Come on," I thought. "Please don't be something bad."

"YOU'RE TELLING ME I HAVE CANCER?"

When I emerged from the fentanyl and midazolam haze, I saw that a nurse had removed my IV line from a vein in my left hand.

There was a little purple bruise where the needle had been. The colonoscopy was done.

I was wearing one of those starchy, pastel-blue hospital gowns. I looked around the room and saw other patients, some sleeping, some skimming celebrity magazines. Smooth jazz played softly in the background, and there were prints of boats and mountains on the walls.

It could have been any recovery room, in any medical facility, in Anytown, USA.

My wife came into focus by my side. The gastroenterologist was ready to see us in his office so a nurse ushered us in and closed the door behind her as she left.

Before the colonoscopy, Dr. K. had been upbeat. We lived in the same town and we both had children in the school district. He had sized me up and suggested maybe it was hemorrhoids or ulcers causing my blood loss. After all, I was young, strong, and healthy.

Now the mood had shifted. He looked down at his desk. There was a quiet moment before he looked up.

"Trevor, you have a mass within your ascending colon, on the right side of your abdomen. It's large—about 9 or 10 centimeters. It's not obstructing your colon yet, but it's close. It's been there for a while." He paused. "We took samples of it for biopsy. You're going to need surgery soon. I can refer you to a surgical oncologist."

Mass. Biopsy. Oncologist.

"Cancer. You're telling me I have cancer?" I asked.

"Yes, almost certainly," Dr. K. said.

What. The. Fuck.

I looked at Sarah. Her mouth had dropped open. We've been together since we were teenagers. My legs turned to rubber.

7

Until that point, there had been nothing remarkable about my health.

I was slightly overweight. I drank an occasional bourbon, but I'd never had a problem with alcohol. I smoked socially for a time in college, then sporadically for a few years after that. My diet was good. I got plenty of exercise.

Yet here I was with a softball-sized tumor in my large intestine and who knows where else in my body. My head spun. Somehow, I gathered myself to ask Dr. K. some questions.

"Can you tell if the cancer has spread beyond the colon?"

"Not sure." He shook his head. "I'll need a CT scan."

"When will we get the results of the biopsy?"

"Within a week," he said.

"Do you see tumors like this in people my age?"

"More and more lately, unfortunately."

The debriefing was over in five minutes. Dr. K. shook our hands. He wished us the best of luck, opened the door, and ushered us out into a world that looked the same, but was suddenly and completely foreign.

We got into our car, reached for each other, and gasped for air. The girls. How on earth were we going to tell the girls?

It was March 22, 2018.

And that is how the cancer journey starts—in a small medical office after a routine procedure, when a nurse shuts a door, and the silence hangs in the air a bit too long.

It starts with a stranger whose job it is to tell people just like me, and families just like ours, that my odds of living essentially come down to a dice roll.

TELLING THE KIDS

For three or four days after my diagnosis, I was calm, cool, and collected. I made the necessary phone calls to my father, mother, brother, other relatives, and friends. It was surreal, like I was talking to them about dinner plans.

"Um, so, I have cancer. We don't know how bad it is yet. We aren't sure what is going to happen, but I'm sure we'll get through it."

Looking back, I remember thinking: Wow, I'm handling this pretty well. I didn't realize that was only because I was in actual physiological shock. My entire life—all the stories I had told myself about my health and longevity and where I fit in the world—had been shattered. I had not even begun to process any of it yet.

One of those nights, Sarah and I sat the girls down at the dining room table. Our plan was to be open and honest but not get into the details. Without a guidebook on how to have this conversation, we did the best we could.

Sage was in 7th grade, a gentle and loving spirit, quiet and shy. She was a beautiful singer, with much more going on in her mind than she was ready to share. Underneath her shyness, though, was a determination to thrive.

Elsie was in 5th grade, full of energy and enthusiasm. When Elsie was in a room, you knew it. She was assertive, playful, and confident, even among adults. She always wanted to make everyone happy.

Both girls were highly sensitive to our emotions. They knew something serious was going on when we sat them down.

"You've heard about cancer, right?" I asked them. "You know it's a disease where a person's cells grow out of control, creating these growths called tumors."

They did know about it, mostly from television shows and advertisements for cancer treatments. Honestly, we had not talked about cancer much at all as a family because we didn't have any close relatives going through it. My own grandparents on my father's side had died of cancer, but that was in old age and long ago.

"Well, I have cancer. It's in my digestive system," I told them. I explained a bit about the large intestine and its function. "I'm going to need surgery so the doctors can remove the cancer. Then I will probably go on medications, called chemotherapy, to make sure all the cancer gets killed."

The girls nodded their heads. We were calm, so they were calm. It must have seemed to them that we had this thing handled, just like we handled everything else. Finally, Elsie spoke up.

"But they are going to get it all, right? They're going to kill all the cancer?"

And here's the point, as a parent facing a life-threatening illness, where you have to make an important choice.

You have to decide if you'll tell them: Yes, the cancer will be all killed and life will be back to normal. Or if you tell them the truth: I don't know.

Now, this is one of the trickiest of all decisions, because no one wants to scare their children. I certainly did not want to scare Sage and Elsie.

But I already knew this about our kids—they would know if we lied to them. And then they would be processing this news alone, in secret, having lost the trust we built over their lifetimes. If we lied, they wouldn't believe us down the road, when the stakes would be even more clear.

So this is what I said: "Yes, the plan is that the doctors will do the surgery and kill all the cancer, and I won't ever have to do anything else. I can't promise you that because we don't know exactly what will happen. But I can promise you this: I will do everything in my power to get rid of this cancer, to be healthy, and to be here for you."

And that was pretty much the conversation. We snuggled up on the couch and watched an episode of *Survivor*. They were content, I think, because I had told them the truth in that moment, and I know they believed me.

I imagined, like any good father, that I would carry them through it.

I had no idea how much they would end up carrying me.

NOT AN OLD MAN'S DISEASE

"Hopefully, this will be about six months of your life. And in a few years it will all seem like a dream," my local oncologist, Dr. Devon Evans, told me following my colon surgery when I was undergoing chemotherapy in the summer of 2018.

The report from my surgery had shown the large mass in my ascending colon was indeed cancerous, along with one lymph node. But the CT scan didn't show anything else to be concerned about.

If only his original prediction had held true.

About 150,000 new patients are diagnosed each year with colorectal cancer, according to the National Cancer Institute. Colorectal cancer is also known as "CRC," the umbrella term for cancer that develops in either the colon or the rectum.

People think it's an "old man's disease," but colorectal cancer is divided nearly equally between men and women, and there has been a disturbing rise among younger adults. A person born in 1990 has double the risk of colon cancer, and four times the risk of rectal cancer, than a person born in 1950.

Many of these young people are otherwise healthy and have no major risk factors, such as poor diet or lack of exercise, leaving scientists at a loss to explain the uptick. Yet we don't often hear about CRC in the news like we hear about other cancers.

If you are diagnosed with colorectal cancer before it metastasizes, in stages I–III, your chances for survival are excellent. At those stages, roughly 70–90 percent of patients will be alive at the five-year mark after diagnosis, depending on individual factors.

For stage IV, though, the prognosis is dismal. Less than 15 percent of stage IV patients are alive at the five-year mark.

Although there has been progress in treatment options, most of the new therapies only extend patients' lives by a period of months, and the five-year survival statistic has not changed significantly in quite some time.

When colorectal cancer spreads, usually it goes to the liver, lungs, and the abdominal cavity and its lining, called the peritoneum. My first CT scan didn't show any metastasis, so I thought my first three months of chemotherapy would get me into the "cured" category.

My second CT scan, in September of 2018, felt like a cruel hoax.

"There is a lesion on your liver," Dr. Evans told us when we met to go over the results. "Looking back at your first scan, it was there back in March, and it has grown. We aren't going to jump to conclusions, but it could be cancer that spread from your colon."

Stage IV cancer. Sarah and I went numb, again. In a single sentence, I had gone from the realm of "most likely to be cured" to "most likely terminal."

I would need to set up appointments with surgeons to see if the liver tumor could be removed. I called my father and asked him to watch Sage and Elsie after school so Sarah and I could have some time to process, which meant sitting in the car again, crying and raging against the news.

By that point, my mental health had already spiraled downward. I was lost in obsessive journaling about my symptoms and constantly researching online about my disease. I was barely engaging with anyone else, even my own family.

When we confirmed that I was a stage IV patient, that broke me.

At night, my dreams were about mazes I couldn't escape and riddles I couldn't solve. I would wake in a sweat, my heart and temples pounding. I felt like a wounded, trapped animal, clawing at my cage.

My medical providers, from those at my oncologist's office and at the hospitals where I received care to my primary care physician, cycled me through a laundry list of medications

14

in an attempt to regain my emotional stability—Ativan, Lexapro, Buspar, Remeron. But my mental health only got worse, to the point of debilitation.

Those were the days spent on my knees in despair. No longer the man of the house, I had been reduced to the man of the living room floor.

CHAPTER 2

HEROES

WE ALL KNOW a variation of this guy: His jaw is swollen twice its normal size. He walks around town wincing in pain, but when anyone asks if he's OK, he says he's fine. You notice that he spends a lot of time alone.

You ask him, "How long has your jaw been hurting?"

"Oh, not that long," he says. "Well, I guess it has been hurting for a while."

"Like, a few months?"

"More like a few years," he admits.

And when you press him, you find out he hasn't been to see a doctor. The excuses are endless: "It's going to cost too much." "I don't trust doctors." "I don't have time." "I'm sure it's nothing." "I can handle it." "I'm not a wimp."

Men tend to ignore the symptoms of health problems not for days or weeks but for years. And when we get injured or sick, we tend to isolate far more often than women.

When facing a cancer diagnosis, men tend to "check out" while women tend to "reach out."

Now of course, this doesn't apply to all men or all women. Every cancer journey is different based on the individual. However, as you will read throughout the chapters of this book, there is a mountain of data, along with countless personal anecdotes, to back up the central premise that men and women respond differently when faced with a life-threatening illness.

These different responses are the result of culture (how we are raised and mentored), combined with biological traits that are products of evolutionary history.

Men are more likely to be diagnosed with cancer at a later stage and have a higher risk of dying, according to the National Cancer Institute and the American Cancer Society.

Why? In large part, it comes down to behavior. Men are less likely to see a doctor for any reason, including cancer screenings. They are less likely to have health insurance or seek second opinions. They smoke, drink alcohol, and take drugs at higher rates than women. And after they are diagnosed with cancer, men are more likely to struggle with social isolation, anxiety, and depression.

With roughly one million new cases of cancer each year for American men, these trends represent a significant public health problem.

"THE GUY PROBLEM"

Dr. Joseph Greer has seen the "guy problem" throughout the course of his two-decade career as a psychologist who counsels cancer patients and their family members. Along with his clinical practice, he is also a researcher.

Greer is program director of the Center for Psychiatric Oncology & Behavioral Sciences, and is co-director of the Cancer Outcomes Research & Education Program at the Massachusetts General Hospital Cancer Center. He is also an associate professor of psychology at Harvard Medical School.

"For men in particular, they want the people around them to know that they are OK and they don't want to cause undue stress. So one reaction is to filter a lot of what they're going through, so they are not sharing openly," Greer said, when I interviewed him on the topic. "That can be very isolating. On top of that, we have this stiff-upper-lip belief that we just have to shoulder it on our own."

Greer said he works to break down those barriers and help his male clients understand that emotional distress during cancer is a common experience, and they can really benefit if they can let their guard down.

"One comment I hear a lot from the guys is this: 'I never would have come to see you if it weren't for my oncologist,'" Greer told me. "But after the first session, they are pretty much sold. They see the benefits."

I've had people ask me why it matters if men isolate when facing cancer. Why should we care if a man decides to check out and go through the cancer diagnosis and treatment on his own?

I tell them there are three major consequences of isolation when facing cancer, and none of them are good.

Mental Health Struggles

Social isolation during cancer and other serious health challenges is connected with an increased risk of anxiety, substance abuse, depression, and suicide.

Relationships

The intensity of emotional and physical stress during cancer magnifies patterns of behavior within relationships. Couples are confronting changing roles and responsibilities. Men often withdraw from relationships with spouses and children because they don't want to cause pain to loved ones. This can cause unintended harm.

Medical Outcomes

Cancer patients who are isolated are at higher risk of dying from cancer versus patients who have social support, according to American Cancer Society research. There are many contributing factors to this. When men isolate, they don't seek the best medical care possible. They don't seek second or third opinions. They don't connect with other patients, who are often the greatest sources of information about doctors and treatment options.

That last point is where I really get a guy's attention. I start with these three reasons for not isolating, and usually that's enough to convince a skeptic.

If you're a man going through cancer, do your best to stay connected to other people and various communities. If you're someone who cares about a man facing the disease, the first and best thing you can do is to make sure he is not isolated.

"THERE ISN'T A PLAYBOOK"

Kevin Gillespie was diagnosed with a rare form of kidney cancer in May of 2018, when he was 35 years old. In the early days of coping with cancer, he remembers that his isolation was fueled by bitterness.

"I started thinking: This was my journey and I have to do this on my own. I didn't care who was there. And that's a shame because I had a lot of friends come visit during that phase of my mental health. And I didn't care. I was just so mad, you know, and I hate that, frankly," he told me. "I'm not a man with many regrets in his life, but I regret not really taking in and being present in those moments more than I was."

Kevin is an acclaimed chef, restaurant owner, and business-man from Georgia who became a breakout star on Bravo's award-winning television series *Top Chef*.

He said he might have remained isolated during cancer, but his public profile made it hard for him to stay hidden in his man cave.

"I felt like the burden had to be shouldered by me and only me, and it's too much to carry by yourself, to be honest with you. It just crushes you. And I was very fortunate that maybe because of my public presence, people knew how to get in touch with me. So I got such a tremendous amount of letters and emails and text messages with encouragement that it made an enormous difference," Kevin said.

One friend in particular, another young cancer patient who ultimately died from the disease, challenged him to evolve his mindset.

"They helped me recognize that in the suffering there was beauty—there was an opportunity coming from it. The fact that they were willing to carry some of my burden for me because they knew that their life was going to be over sooner than later. That just completely changed me," Kevin said.

"I realized that I had to get better as fast as I could safely," he said. "Because I had an obligation now to everyone else who was going through this, to help people understand that it is OK to go through all of those phases. It is OK to be angry, frustrated, and sad."

"There isn't a playbook that just works for everybody," Kevin told me. "But the cornerstone truth for everyone is that the journey is easier if you let the people who want to take it with you come along. If you let them help carry the load, it'll be a lot better."

―――――――――――

IN MY MAN CAVE

I wasn't ready to come out of my man cave in the fall of 2018. Not even close.

I remember thinking it would be so much easier if I were a hermit, living on my own in the northern Maine woods. I envisioned myself in a cabin up by Mount Katahdin. I could be sick in solitude there, no longer a burden to Sarah and the girls.

At one point that fall, I was experiencing such bad abdominal pain that Sarah basically forced me to go to a doctor for some hands-on therapy for my belly.

After five minutes of working on me, the doctor took her hands away and sat upright on her stool. She asked me, slowly and deliberately: "Trevor, do you want to be here?"

I knew she wasn't asking if I wanted to be in her office, receiving therapy.

She was asking if I wanted to live.

The tears I had been holding back streamed down my cheeks. I took a long time to reflect on this question, one that no one had asked before. I wasn't having suicidal thoughts, but it was true that my will to live was weaker than it had ever been.

"Yes," I said finally. "I want to be here for my family. But I don't want to be a burden anymore. I feel like I've failed them."

Looking back, it's not a surprise that I felt like a failure.

Cancer patients are supposed to inspire us, right? The male cancer patients shown in the media are relentlessly brave and optimistic. In magazines, TV segments, on book covers, and in our social media feeds you see them caring for their families, working full time, and participating in 5K fundraisers, all while slaying cancer at every turn.

To put it mildly, I didn't look like that. I was in my room, sick from chemo and depression, while my dad mowed the lawn and my friends stacked the firewood.

As American men, we're conditioned by our culture to "man up" when a challenge comes along. We're taught to rub dirt on our wounds, saddle up, toughen up, don't complain, and don't talk about it. We're supposed to tackle challenges on our own.

Even in 2022, we still raise boys to numb and bury their feelings—to be rugged individuals. Through advertising, the media, and the role models available to us in real life, men are conditioned to be tough guys, not whole human beings. The emotional fallout is devastating. I've watched too many friends slide into patterns of abuse, broken relationships, and destructive addiction.

Fortunately for me, I grew up in a household where it was OK to have the whole range of human feelings and to share them. I had permission to be competitive, while also having permission to cry openly, to hug the people close to me and tell them, "I love you." But that environment in my house only went so far.

As a boy growing up in the 1980s, most of my heroes were larger-than-life, macho guys.

He-Man, G.I. Joe, Luke Skywalker—those were my toys. And my other heroes were sports stars like José Canseco, Roger Clemens, Larry Bird, and Michael Jordan; action stars like Arnold Schwarzenegger and Bruce Willis; and wrestlers like Hulk Hogan.

For starters, none of those guys would ever show weakness. Those guys would never get cancer, and if they somehow did, they would crush it just like they crushed any opponents who got in their way.

When you get to be an adult, you look back and see that those hero narratives didn't reflect the full human experience. They were real life on steroids, sometimes literally. Most of us understand, at some point, that our childhood heroes are just characters, created by marketers to entertain us and sell products to kids.

But those early imprints provided me with some of my first ideas about what it means to be a man and how a man should behave. And those first imprints are sticky as hell.

So what happens to the American man, one who has been taught there is no hurdle he can't handle on his own, when a challenge comes along that he can't simply fix?

What happens when he gets cancer?

In a word: Shame.

The man who trusted his body feels betrayed by it. The man who had developed confidence in his environment feels suddenly and irrevocably lost. He's facing a killer disease that he knows nothing about, without the language or tools to fight it. Now he's reduced to being a "patient" at the mercy of doctors, insurers, and the health care system.

If you ever imagined yourself as He-Man, like I did, cancer wasn't in the script.

"WE'RE SUPPOSED TO BE TOUGH"

J.J. Singleton, 34, was raised in the rough-and-tough culture of football in rural North Carolina. His father played at Virginia Tech, his uncle played at the collegiate level, and J.J. played at a small college before too many concussions forced him to give up the sport.

After football ended, J.J. went to work for his uncle, who owned convenience stores, car washes, and hardware stores.

But when J.J.'s athletic career was over, there was a hole in his life in his 20s that he tried to fill with drinking, partying, and overeating.

"I just wanted to have fun with my friends. On college-football Saturdays, I would wake up and start drinking until I passed out, eating a lot of pizza and wings in between," he said.

In 2015 he was promoted to operations manager and was ready to change his life. He changed his diet and joined a CrossFit gym, working out there during his lunch break. He dropped weight quickly and started to feel like his old self again.

It was less than a year later when he first felt a throbbing pain in his left flank. He was already signed up for an upcoming CrossFit competition, so he pushed through the pain, even as it got more intense. After the competition, his body crashed. He couldn't eat or drink without abdominal pain, and he wasn't having regular bowel movements.

"I would look up the symptoms online, and cancer was always listed at the bottom. I was like, 'That ain't right. That ain't gonna happen,'" he said. "I knew something was wrong, but I still didn't want to go to the doctor because I didn't even have a regular doctor in my 20s. I didn't like money coming out of my check to pay for health insurance. But one night, when I went to my mom's house, she was like, 'You've gotta go to the doctor tomorrow. You're turning gray!'"

In September of 2015, at age 27, J.J. was diagnosed with stage IV colorectal cancer.

Since that time, he has undergone more than 10 major surgeries and more than 100 rounds of chemotherapy and immunotherapy. During one brutal stretch, he was on a feeding tube for 450 days.

Like Kevin Gillespie, J.J. often experienced a pull toward isolation. His mom, dad, step-parents, and grandparents were supportive all the way. But other guys he thought were his friends vanished after his diagnosis. There were times when J.J. felt consumed with rage, unable to understand why he was facing cancer just when he was getting his health, and life, back on track.

"I didn't want to share my depression or the sadness that came because, you know, I grew up a man. We're supposed to be tough, and not show that vulnerable side. So I kept my emotions down," he said. "That's why I help as many people as I can, especially younger people going through cancer, because I get it. I want to bring acknowledgement to all the layers of cancer."

Over the past few years, J.J. has emerged as a leader for other young people facing cancer, by finding the courage to share his struggles along with his successes.

J.J. blogs and posts on social media about his ongoing battles with anxiety, depression, and PTSD. He has written about his suicidal thoughts, and the people who've surrounded him with love—who carry him through.

> *Some days are hard and make me wish for 1 day I*
>   *could be free from it all.*
>
> *Free from the stress*
>
> *Free from the anxiety*
>
> *Free from the PTSD*
>
> *Free from the mental exhaustion*
>
> *Free from the pain*
>
> *Free from the physical effects that control life*
>
> *Free from the weight it places on me*
>
> *Free from the regret of putting this on people*
>
> *Free from treatments*
>
> *Free from cancer*
>
> *24 hours of the life I knew for 27 years is all I'd*
>   *ask for.*
>
>   – J.J. Singleton

Nearly every day, J.J. receives messages from other patients and survivors who identify with his emotions and his writing. They thank him for his transparency. In some instances, they have thanked him for saving their lives.

"Once the cancer came back and it really started affecting me mentally, I knew it was gonna be this way pretty much for the rest of my life," J.J. said. "That's why I was like, 'I gotta be open about it, and if I can help one person it's all worth it.'"

CHAPTER 3

THE PANERA INCIDENT

IN ADVANCE OF this particular tale, I apologize to the good people of Panera Bread company. I enjoy your soups, sandwiches, and bottomless coffee refills.

It's not your fault that some of your patrons are heartless jerks.

In November of 2018, I was getting ready for surgery to remove at least one, possibly more, tumors from my liver. The liver is an essential organ, with plenty of blood supply designed to remove waste products and toxins from the bloodstream. That makes it an ideal environment for metastatic cancer (cancer that has spread from its original location).

Up to 30 percent of colorectal cancer patients will have the disease spread to their livers at some point, and that's exactly what happened to me.

Sarah and I interviewed two surgeons in Maine and one in Boston. Ultimately, we decided to go with Dr. Lisa Rutstein, a highly skilled and compassionate surgeon at Central Maine Medical Center.

The goal was simple: Remove the liver tumors and get me to the point of being cancer-free, hopefully for good.

The surgery itself, however, would not be simple. Dr. Rutstein, along with other doctors and a medical team, would need to open my entire abdomen, roll my liver over, and carefully cut out a wedge of tissue containing my tumor. They would then ultrasound the liver and check for any other tumors.

For most metastatic cancers, including colorectal, the gold standard for reaching NED (No Evidence of Disease) is usually a combination of systemic therapy, such as chemo, and surgery. For some disease types, the acronym NED has replaced the word "remission." Both terms mean there is no detectable cancer in the body.

Dr. Rutstein didn't pull any punches. My chances for recurrence would be high after the surgery, she told us. Once cancer gets to stage IV, when it's in your blood and your lymphatic system, it almost always comes back. But I was relatively young, otherwise healthy, and physically strong. We were ready to take this shot.

I should remind you here that I was in a dark place, mentally, in the weeks leading up to this surgery.

For the first time in a long time, I decided to actually get out of the house....

Yep, look at me go. I drive to some shops, thinking I might get a few presents for Sarah and the girls. I know I'll be out of commission for a while after surgery, probably through Christmas.

While I'm out shopping, I pop into Panera for lunch, order a grilled cheese sandwich and tomato soup, and sit down next to four men who appear to be in their 50s.

As if my luck weren't bad enough, these guys are talking, intensely, about cancer.

"It's proven that cancer is a psychological disease. People get it because they have a psychological roadblock they haven't dealt with," this one guy says. "So when you remove the roadblock, you heal your cancer. There are lots of books on this."

Oh, shit. This is not really happening. I feel my face getting hot.

Another guy picks up where his friend left off.

"I agree. A friend of mine had cancer and she used yoga to clear her chakras because they were blocked. It's about getting unstuck where you are stuck."

At that point, I'm boiling. I visualize throat punching one of the guys, then upending the table in a dramatic heave, covering all four of them in their lunches.

Instead, I turn to them and smile.

"Excuse me, guys, I'm a stage IV cancer patient. In a few weeks I'm going into a surgery we hope will save my life.

Just overhearing your conversation, I couldn't help but think, maybe you want to come over to my house and explain to my 13-year-old and 11-year-old daughters how I caused my own cancer because of psychological road-blocks."

They stare at me, mouths agape. Maybe they think I'm actually going to upend the table. After a long pause, one of them stumbles through a reply.

"We didn't mean...that was not meant to.... Sorry if we offended you. Is there anything we can do to help?"

"Look, this is a free country," I say. "You can believe whatever you want to believe. I'm not here to tell you how to think or what to say. I just want you to understand that when you are in a public place like this, you might want to think about your conversations and how they might feel to a person like me. I don't need that kind of judgment right now."

And then I stand up and walk away.

TOXIC POSITIVITY

The Panera incident was my first, and certainly not my last, experience with what would become my ultimate cancer peeve—toxic positivity.

It's the mindset that all will work out in your favor if you wish it to be true, and there is no room for "negative" thoughts and feelings.

In the realm of Cancerland, toxic positivity often happens when well-intentioned people—sometimes even those who are close to you—feel compelled to let you know that a cure is right around the corner, through the power of the mind, spirit, carrot juice, or some combination of all of the above.

Usually this unsolicited advice comes from cancer muggles (people who've never personally experienced cancer but think they know everything about it).

"Just think positive." "Attitude is everything." "Don't give it power over you."

These are some of the pithy expressions that you hear every-where when you have cancer. I'm surprised we don't get a box of them in the mail within a week of diagnosis.

No matter what is said, the message is clear: You, the pa-tient, have the power for self healing.

I get it. I really do. Cancer is scary. It is among the scariest of all health problems. People want to believe, especially in the United States, that we're in full control of our individual destinies. They want to believe that if we become ill, then we must have done something to deserve it. And by the power of positivity, we can chart our own course back to health.

This belief has deep roots in both religious and secular dog-ma, and, wow, is it pervasive.

33

Kate Bowler is an author and an associate professor of American religious history at Duke University. Like me, she is a young-onset, stage IV colorectal cancer survivor. She was diagnosed in 2015 at age 35.

In her book *Everything Happens for a Reason, and Other Lies I've Loved*, Bowler recounts her own diagnosis and treatment in the context of her studies of "the prosperity gospel." Essentially, the prosperity gospel is a Christian theology centered on this idea: If you live simply and in devotion to God, you will be rewarded with health and good fortune in this lifetime. Bowler explains it further as she struggles with the concept when facing her own cancer.

> To believers in the prosperity gospel, surrender sounds like defeat. They write books with titles like Deal with It! *to remind readers that there is nothing so difficult that God cannot accomplish it, and that you, sir or ma'am, had better get cracking. There are no setbacks, just setups. There are no trials, just tests of character. Tragedies are simply opportunities to claim a bigger, better miracle.*

I thought about Bowler and her book when, not long after my lovely lunch at Panera, I went to deposit some checks at my local bank.

The bank teller happened to glance at a folder that I had set on the counter. I had scribbled "Cancer surgery—Notes" on it.

"Are you having surgery?" she asked as she scanned the checks, one by one, into the computer.

I nodded.

"I had a cancer scare once," she said. "I wasn't feeling good so I went and saw some doctors. They were thinking maybe I had cancer. At first I was pretty shaken, but I knew what I had to do. I went home; I closed my eyes; and all I thought about was NOT having cancer. I visualized that nothing was there. So the next time I went back to the doctors, they did a scan, and—just like I KNEW—there was nothing there. I didn't have cancer! You should do the same thing. You might not need surgery," she said.

I stood there and stared at her without showing emotion. As she handed me my receipt, I said "Thank you." And when I walked outside, I felt gutted.

How could someone think it's OK to counsel a cancer patient like that, without even being asked? I know the answer. They think they're being helpful. I can categorically tell you: This guidance is not helpful.

Imagine a bank teller offering this advice to a person with a spinal cord injury: "Just be positive. Visualize your spinal cord whole and healthy."

Or suggesting to a person with type 1 diabetes: "Attitude is everything! Just think about your pancreas working properly and that'll happen for you."

For other physical illnesses, you don't hear that kind of stuff much outside of the most hardcore evangelical settings. But with cancer, there seem to be no filters or limits.

As cancer patients, we're made to feel that something we did, something we ate, something we thought (or our overall poor mindset) caused our cancer. If we would just think the right way, or pray the right way, or fix our chakras, we would heal ourselves. We are routinely lectured and shamed. Somehow, it's culturally acceptable to shame us.

———————

FULL EMOTIONS, LIMITED POWER

Most cancer patients grapple with fears about their disease. I certainly have had my share of grappling sessions.

"What if the scan report or the blood work isn't good?" "What if my tumors have grown, and there are more tumors in my liver...and possibly my lungs?" "What am I going to tell my wife and kids?"

When you've had lots of scans, and lots of bad news, these fears are the sticky residue of emotional trauma.

Whenever I make this admission—that I'm nervous and having some scary thoughts—I can hear the whispering voices of cultural judgment.

Talk about a burden.

Dr. Greer, the psychologist from Massachusetts General Hospital, describes this as the "pervasive culture of positive thinking in the cancer world."

"The fact is, that is not people's experience," Dr. Greer said. "There is a range of emotions and thoughts that come along with the cancer experience, and that's normal and healthy. We shouldn't just ignore those."

Toxic positivity reigns in cancer literature, in the magazines and books that get top display in the bookstores, in podcasts, and radio interviews. The thing is, if reaching a cure was as easy as willing our cells back into good behavior, I don't think 600,000 Americans would have died from cancer in 2020.

Here's the tricky part about positivity for me as a patient.

I actually do believe I can improve my health through positivity and taking care of my mind. Science has proven this to be true, and breakthroughs continue to be made regarding the mind-body connection.

But that power is limited. I don't believe I have omnipotent control of my health.

Far wiser and more capable thinkers than I have tried, and failed, to manifest a cure for themselves. This is why the writer, philosopher, and farmer Wendell Berry wisely reminds us that we are creations, not creators.

It's normal and sane to be afraid. In fact, fear is perhaps the

37

best evidence of my humanity. It means I want more time on this earth with my family and friends.

So when the anxiety rises and the dark thoughts come, I try not to push them away. Instead, I get right up close to them. I examine them, feeling compassion for myself. And when they pass, which they always do, I appreciate the light more than ever.

All of those emotions are vital when facing a life-threatening illness. We are healthier when we access our full range of emotions, when we allow ourselves—without guilt—to cry, scream, rage, and yes, even wallow at times. We are unhealthy when we suppress those thoughts and feelings, when we don't allow ourselves to be fully human.

If you are a fellow patient and the "all positive, all the time" mindset works for you, I wish you all the best.

I realized early in my journey that it wasn't a fit for me. I had to find a different approach. I have latched on to a piece of wisdom from the Buddhist tradition: Be open to all experiences and outcomes but attached to none.

I'm hopeful for great results, and I imagine those will happen for me, but I don't cling desperately to that outcome. I acknowledge the possibility of receiving difficult news.

The truth is, most of us are just doing the best we can to be healthy, to live long lives with our families with the resources we have on hand and with the cards we were dealt.

If you have people in your life who don't allow you to feel all the feels of cancer, especially the uncomfortable ones, tell them to stop.

And if they won't, maybe it's time to find some new friends.

CHAPTER 4

MY SHAWSHANK MOMENT

IF YOU HAVEN'T seen the movie *The Shawshank Redemption*, do yourself a favor and watch it.

Tim Robbins plays Andy Dufresne, a man falsely accused of murdering his wife. While serving a life sentence in Shawshank Prison, Andy becomes fast friends with another man convicted of murder, Ellis Boyd "Red" Redding, played by the legendary actor Morgan Freeman.

SPOILER ALERT! The turning point in the movie happens when Andy makes the decision to take control of his destiny, exact revenge on the corrupt prison warden, break out of Shawshank, and head to a beach town in Mexico.

"I guess it comes down to a simple choice, Red," Andy says. "Get busy living, or get busy dying."

At some point, most of us face that fork in the road. There's no going back, and the way forward will be down one road... or the other.

My Shawshank moment happened around Christmas 2018.

I was home, recovering from liver surgery. Dr. Rutstein and her team had managed to remove the metastatic tumor from the dome of my liver. They didn't find any other cancer when they were in there, but my recovery was brutal.

I left the hospital with a drain tube, which allowed residual blood and related fluid to drain from my abdomen, through a tube that came out of my lower belly, and into a rubber bulb. I would wear sweatpants every day and keep the bulb in my pocket, emptying it a few times a day.

To get the fluid to drain properly, I would need to "strip" the drain tube, which meant pinching it so the fluid would be drawn out. Some people say this stripping doesn't bother them, but for me, it hurt like hell. The pain rippled up through my insides all the way into my diaphragm.

For most of December, as my internal and external wounds were healing, my abdomen felt like it was on fire. I would lie on the couch during the day; night sweats and vivid, gruesome dreams kept me up at night.

My personal prison—anxiety and depression from that summer and fall—had not improved. If anything, I felt even more like a prisoner. I might not have said it to anyone at the time, but I was convinced that I was a failure, and I was going to die.

While I was going through this physical and emotional darkness, I felt utterly alone. I had spoken with a few other cancer patients over the prior six months, but I was not close with them. I was surrounded by helpful friends and family, but we might as well have been a million miles apart. In my mind, no one could understand what I was feeling. No one could relate.

My wife Sarah's frustration, understandably, was growing by the day. For months, she had been carrying the family by herself, taking the girls where they needed to go, helping with their homework, doing the meals and the cleaning. It was all on her shoulders. I could see the steam building up inside her but felt helpless to do anything about it.

My identity was shattered, and I could not imagine any possible way to get it back. I had gone from being a good-natured, outward-thinking person, someone who always thinks of his family and friends first, to a person who was obsessed solely with his own dire circumstances.

When I wasn't staring off into space, I was searching Google for everything related to my disease—scientific studies, statistics, patient experiences, drug summaries, descriptions of side effects, pretty much anything I could find about colorectal cancer…and none of it was positive.

My depression was affecting everyone in the family. Sage and Elsie would take turns snuggling up to me while watching TV shows. It was their way of trying to pull me out.

One day, Elsie found an old family photo of the four of us and pasted it on her brightly colored drawing of a hot air balloon. We are all smiling and happy in the photo, which was taken years before cancer. She wrote the captions: "HOPE," and "Up, up, and away!"

THE BREAKING POINT

That's when the breaking point happened. After the girls were tucked in for the night, Sarah and I got into bed. She sat up and looked at me.

"Things need to change," she said. "This is a nightmare. My worst nightmare. I feel like even if you survive cancer, we are losing you. You have to feel better. I need you to feel better."

I hung my head, feeling my eyes burning from the tears that were coming.

We had been together for so long and had built our entire lives together—yet in that mix of depression and shame, I had nothing to offer her.

"Do you want to leave? Do you want me to leave?" I asked.

"No," she said. "You're not getting what I'm trying to tell you."

She stood up in the space between our bed and her wooden dresser. Her eyes welled up. She was trembling and had a desperate look.

"You can't leave, and I don't want you to leave," she said, raising her voice. "I want you to get better. We need you here with us—the real you."

Her words hung there, and my mind raced to fill the void. The rest of the house was quiet.

"I'm trying.... I'm trying.... I don't know what to do," I said, feeling my panic through the pounding of my heart.

"The thought of not being here for the girls is killing me," I told her. " I can't do this. I can't get over it. If I die, they're just going to remember me sick during chemo, with tubes from the surgeries, lying on the couch all day. I'm afraid they're going to just remember me as sick."

She took that in for a long moment. We sat in silence. Then she looked at me—I know that look when she wants to say something but isn't sure if I'm ready to hear it.

"Say it. It's OK, I want you to say what you have to say," I told her.

By this point I was sobbing. Sarah got real still and calm.

"I'm not worried they're going to remember you as sick," she said. "I'm worried they're going to remember you as sad."

Damn. I had been on the verge of cracking open for a long time, and that sentence was the sledgehammer.

Sarah was right. That's not who I am. I'm not a sad person. Before cancer, I had normal times of sadness of course, but I was a positive and playful person, always encouraging others. And I was especially joyous with my wife and our girls.

When that sledgehammer of a sentence hit me, I visualized the two roads stretching out ahead of us, and I knew in that moment that I needed to choose one.

I could continue down the road of grief, fear, anxiety, and depression, and the girls would remember me as sad, just like Sarah said.

Or I could get busy living.

GET BUSY LIVING

How many guys are lucky enough to have a wife like Sarah, and daughters like Sage and Elsie? I don't think very many.

At rock bottom, when all I was doing was pushing them away, they were bold and brave enough to love me through it.

Not only did they refuse to let me leave, they believed in me, even in my brokenness. I use the word "gratitude" all the time, but it hardly captures the emotions that I have in my heart for these three humans.

Sarah saved me that night. She could've easily walked out the door; others certainly would've taken that easier route. She might tell you it's because she's the most stubborn person in the world. I will tell you it's because that stubbornness can come in handy when it comes to love.

So we sat there for a few minutes. I composed myself, taking some long, deep breaths. I looked her in the eyes.

"I hear you. And I am with you," I said. "Here's the deal. It took me a long time to get to this place, so I'm not going to be able to dig out of this overnight. I wish I could snap my fingers and make that happen, but it's not how this is going to work."

"I'm going to make you a promise," I said. "I'm going to do everything in my power to regain my mental health and get back to that point where I'm living with joy and engagement and purpose."

"Whether I live one more year, or 40 more years, this is my promise to you, and it starts now," I said.

It was a conscious decision and a simple promise, made when I had absolutely no idea how I was going to fulfill it.

―――――――――

ASKING FOR HELP

I knew I couldn't do this alone.

When I was standing at the bottom of that mental-health pit, the first and most important step I took was to admit I needed help.

For me, and a lot of men I know, reaching out and asking for help is not a comfortable place. It doesn't feel like a position of strength. We don't even like to ask for directions, let alone admit that we are broken and in need of help to mend. But what we fail to realize is the fact that there are life-and-death consequences when we don't reach out for help.

For many problems in life, the attitude of can-do individualism is not inherently a weakness. It's perfectly appropriate for a guy to tackle a home improvement project, for example, on his own.

The trouble is, the problem of cancer—and the impossibly heavy baggage that gets heaped on patients during the journey—is not like the problem of a broken pipe.

When a male cancer patient is going through diagnosis and treatment, he does not realize that his chances of survival go down when he takes on the challenges by himself. So he turns to his old patterns, the lessons he learned from those old heroes, and he pushes everyone away. "I'm fine," he says, when he is not at all fine.

Dr. Dianne Shumay is a cancer psychologist who has worked as director of psycho-oncology at the University of California, San Francisco (UCSF) Helen Diller Family Comprehensive Cancer Center. She talked to me about how critical it is for men facing cancer to seek outside help.

"The men I have treated bring the same concerns as anyone facing the stress, uncertainty, and life impacts of cancer. Still, they are showing up less often than women to support groups and individual therapy," Shumay said. "It's documented that men with cancer bring distress about their role functioning as dads, husbands, or on the job. They also bring distress about sexual functioning, as cancer brings a lot of loss in that area. And it is documented that men may see asking for help with these issues as weak."

The team at the UCSF cancer center has tried different strategies to engage men with therapy and other resources. Men-only writing and music groups have been successful, as has a group that combines educational sessions with meals and social time for male cancer patients along with their partners and spouses.

"It is my wish that men with cancer seek and receive the support they need, and that access is not blocked by programs that don't serve men or aren't inviting," Dr. Shumay said. "There are many stereotypes of a man in therapy, or of a man who rejects therapy, but for the guys whom I have treated, they brought to the sessions deep spiritual striving, heartbreaking grief and loss, a determined sense of purpose, their desire to discern their right path, and an ability to love that, frankly, at times has renewed my own sense of optimism about the world."

THE DEMPSEY CENTER

Thanks to Sarah's intervention, I was ready to accept help. My pride took a backseat—all the way back.

I remembered a recommendation that I had received from my amazing oncology nurses when I was going through chemotherapy. They encouraged me to meet people and engage in courses at the Cancer Community Center in South Portland, about a 20-minute drive from our home in Maine.

That community center would soon merge with the Dempsey Center, which was founded in 2008 by the actor Patrick Dempsey, who grew up in Maine.

Much of the world knows Patrick for his iconic roles on TV and in films. To me, he is a real-life hero who has made life better for cancer patients and their families.

Patrick's mother, Amanda Dempsey, lived for 17 years with metastatic ovarian cancer. She was well known for her courage and resilience. Patrick and other members of the family were grateful for the treatment she received at Central Maine Medical Center in Lewiston, but they felt there was a gap in holistic care.

The Dempsey Center was established to provide holistic health services, supporting mental health, nutrition, exercise, massage, reiki, acupuncture, and programs for families—all provided at no cost to clients.

Soon after my breaking-point conversation with Sarah, I visited the Dempsey Center's website and looked at the menu of classes. I had no idea what I was looking for, but I knew I needed to go to something that day. One of the classes was called "Guided Meditation."

After another ten minutes of self doubt, I convinced myself to drive to South Portland....

I'm trembling when I write my name on the Welcome sheet at the front desk. I walk to the designated room and stand in the doorway. The meditation leader is a young woman, probably in her late 20s, with long blonde hair and a pleasant smile. Seated in a circle of chairs are six or seven older women, ranging in age from their 50s to 70s. Most of them wear scarves, covering their hair loss.

They turn and look at me, the giant in the doorframe. They are clearly bewildered or bemused. (Not many men, apparently, attend the guided meditation class.) They don't say anything right away, but I imagine they think I'm there to fix the A/C unit or swap out some furniture.

I introduce myself. "I'm Trevor. I live in Cape Elizabeth. I have a wife and two young daughters. I have stage IV colon cancer... and I could use some help."

The instructor pulls another chair into the circle for me, and the group warms up to me right away. Yes, I'm a man, and I have another version of this hideous disease, but those differences don't matter here; I'm one of them.

We go around the circle making introductions, and the class begins. We close our eyes and take a visit, via meditation, to a beach. I feel the sand and hear the surf. For that fleeting time, I walk away from cancer. When the meditation is over, we all regain our senses and check in with each other.

They are all looking at me. They probably know before I do: The dam is about to break. The burning sensation hits my eyes, and my tears flow.

One of the women shows up on my right side and puts a hand on my shoulder. Another woman does the same on my left side.

"It's OK," they tell me. "Let it out."

And for the next 15 minutes or so, I bawl my freaking eyes out.

I tell them about Sarah, Sage, and Elsie, and about my anger, my fears, my sadness. I tell them all of it. And the whole time they hold me and they nod yes, again and again. I feel loved and seen completely. Because they know. Because they have been exactly where I am. For the first time in more than six months of hell, I have found my people.

"HANG ON, TREVOR"

After the breakthrough crying session with the amazing breast-cancer ladies, I was hooked on the Dempsey Center. I went to as many classes as I could. I exchanged emails and phone numbers with other patients. I even met a few other guys.

Since this was 2019, before the coronavirus pandemic, I

started attending an in-person support group on Wednesday evenings.

The universe then sent another hero into my life, my one-on-one therapist Patti. During those first few sessions, when Patti closed the door and we sat down, she was holding a broken person in her hands. The floodgates for my tears had opened, and it didn't seem they were ever going to stop. At times I felt panicky.

Patti was not fazed. She provided calm, steady, empathetic guidance. I told her that I was never going to make it out of my mental-health pit. She assured me that I would. I told her I was a failure to my family. She assured me I wasn't.

"Hang on, Trevor. Be patient, and be kind to yourself," she would say. "This place that you are in, you will not be there forever. You are getting through it; you are showing up, doing the work…and you're doing it beautifully."

I didn't think my ugly crying was beautiful in any way.

But I kept reminding myself to trust her. This wasn't her first rodeo. I'm not the only cancer patient to grieve the loss of the life I had before, and over her 20-plus years in the field, she had counseled hundreds of us. Her wealth of experience, and her spirit, were the perfect match for me.

By trusting Patti and the people at the Dempsey Center, my recovery was happening, even when I didn't necessarily see it. There were days when I was scheduled to go to a class, or go to a support group, and I just couldn't bring myself to go. But then the next time I would make it until I stopped missing sessions.

My mental health recovery wasn't linear or predictable. I would have a great day, and think I had turned a huge corner, only to retreat and crumble the next day. The pace felt excruciatingly slow. But I knew I was making progress and I had the right people in my life to help me, so I needed to trust the process, even if it felt like walking a tightrope, with a blindfold on...and no safety net.

"BEST DAY POSSIBLE"

It was during those Wednesday evening group counseling sessions that I met another role model, Lona, and learned the phrase "Best Day Possible."

Lona was the matriarch of that group, which usually had about seven or eight participants. We would take turns sharing about what was going on with our cancer and other aspects of our lives, most of all our emotional health.

Lona was in her early 60s, a long-term survivor of a rare neuroendocrine cancer that filled her abdomen up with tumors. She had gone through tons of treatment and what we called "the mother of all surgeries"—her surgeons had removed the disease in her abdomen along with multiple organs and pieces of organs. In short, Lona is a badass. The most compassionate, wise, and kind type of badass.

Although Lona had been disease-free for years, she would still attend the group counseling sessions at the Dempsey Center, mostly because she could be that calm, helpful presence for those of us who were freaking out and losing our shit. Lona was one of my first mentors to teach me about living while going through cancer. She would tell us that in all of the turmoil, we cannot forget to breathe, to play, to love, even when our lives might not be as long as we had hoped. I wasn't ready to absorb that lesson right away, but Lona planted the seed.

At the end of every session, Lona would encourage all of us: "I hope that tomorrow you will have the best day possible."

The word "possible" was intentional. It was Lona's way of telling us that our best day possible might be different from what our best days looked like before cancer. We probably wouldn't go out and run a marathon, climb a mountain, or connect with everyone we had ever cared about.

Best Day Possible is all about doing what you can, where you are, within the limitations of your current situation.

As a cancer patient, maybe your best day possible is getting dressed, taking a shower, or eating a few eggs and toast without vomiting. Maybe it's sending one email or letter to a close friend. Maybe it's a walk around the house.

Learning this phrase, and understanding its meaning, helped relieve some of the pressure I'd been feeling because I wasn't accomplishing much beyond simply surviving.

Lona's message was that all of us sitting in that circle were going through a major, ongoing trauma, physically and mentally, so it's OK to have realistic expectations and to celebrate our successes, even when they might look small to outsiders.

It wasn't fair for us to compare our lives with cancer to the lives we'd lived before our diagnoses and treatments.

Living your Best Day Possible is within the reach of everyone, and I'll always be thankful to Lona for that gift.

CHAPTER 5

WHAT COURAGE REALLY LOOKS LIKE

CANCER TRIED TO drown me.

It was a cold river that rose up far above the banks, plucked me from my pleasant dreams, took me down into the raging current, and smashed me again and again into the rocks.

I choked and flailed and blacked out. I cried out for mercy, for the sake of my wife and kids. I pleaded with the universe, Mother Nature, or whatever gods might listen.

In the early portion of 2019, after my Shawshank moment with Sarah, while I was reaching out for help, I still felt like that frantic swimmer swept up in the ice-cold water whose only instinct is to fight like hell against the current.

I thought if I swam hard enough and long enough, I could get back upstream, back to safety—to that place before cancer.

That's when another helper came into my life, with the right guidance at the right time. Technically, Kate was my physical therapist. I began seeing her for hands-on therapy to help alleviate the pain from my surgical adhesions, the 12-inch scar from liver surgery, and the smaller scar from colon surgery.

In truth, Kate is a healer in the best definition of the word. She bonds instantly with people going through trauma and knows what they need. She does talk therapy while providing manual therapy—and she is insanely intuitive.

"Trevor," she would say, "you are fighting so hard to go back upstream. I want to help you see that you can't get back there. You are in the current, and your only option is to stop struggling and face downstream. I know it's scary, I know you didn't ask for this, but there is no going back to your life before."

The truth of her words were clear, even while I kept flailing.

But I continued to protest.

"I think I can turn downstream, but I'm struggling with my shame," I told her. It was the shame that was relentless. At that time, I was convinced that all cancer patients, except for me of course, handled their diagnosis and treatments with grace and courage. You know, those 5K runners and top fundraisers. They were all crushing it. And here I was, debilitated, letting my family down.

"I'm a mess. I'm failing them," I told her.

"You're being way too hard on yourself. You're not going to be able to understand this now," she said, "but you are exactly where you need to be."

"Courage doesn't always look like what you think it should look like," she said.

And then she told me a story.

One of her physical therapy clients, many years ago, was an elderly man who served in the US Army infantry during the invasion of Normandy in 1944. This man spoke to Kate about his experiences as a soldier and his complex feelings of gratitude and guilt because he had survived when so many of his friends had been killed.

Upon returning home to the States, finding employment, and starting a family, this man enjoyed being a hands-on father; he loved getting on the floor and playing with his kids. But there was one task as a parent that he could not do. He could not change his children's diapers. It wasn't because he didn't want to. It was because the smell of feces triggered in him a trauma so deep that he could not face it.

During the Normandy invasion, when his unit's boat was approaching the beach under heavy German artillery and gunfire, the soldiers were shaking. Some were vomiting, some were crying, a few had soiled themselves. Even as their bodies responded to the likelihood of death by enemy fire, those men still stormed the beach, for their mission and for their love of their brothers beside them.

"Were those men not courageous?" Kate asked me.

"Sometimes courage is messy and ugly and it doesn't look like the movies. It doesn't look like you might want it to," she said. "Courage is not the absence of fear. It is showing up and pressing forward, even when you are most afraid."

"You have plenty of courage, Trevor," she said, "You just need to see it in yourself."

That soldier's story had become part of Kate's story, and from that moment on, it became part of my story, too.

War analogies are a controversial topic in cancer circles. Some patients embrace the similarities and the military language. Others don't want any part of that. For me, I embrace it to a point. With all of my surgeries, scars, and my mortality right in my face because of my dismal prognosis, I absolutely think of myself as a warrior. That said, when I die, if anyone says I "lost the battle" feel free to kick them in the shins for me.

The story of the soldier resonated with every fiber of my being. No other story has felt so freeing. Finally, I could look at myself and see a man who had been crushed, but who was showing up and doing the work.

Before leaving Kate's office that day, I ran my hand across my scars a few times. I looked at myself in the mirror and whispered, "You're a badass."

CULTIVATING MY WARRIOR SPIRIT

Once I started putting the shame behind me, by spring of 2019, the time had come for me to start cultivating my warrior spirit.

My open heart had never been an issue. I have always been a deeply sensitive person, tapped into all of my emotions. But if I was going to be fully equipped to cope with cancer over the course of months and (hopefully) years, I needed to unleash my version of my inner alpha mentality. Let me be clear, I'm not talking about being a jerk or toxic masculinity.

When I talk about "going alpha" I'm talking about refusing to be a victim, getting assertive, taking charge of my circumstances, being accountable, and finding people who will walk the road with me.

Jocko Willink gave me all of that, and I've never even met the guy. Jocko is a retired Navy SEAL commander, with childhood roots in Connecticut and my home state of Maine. In 2006, he was commander of a SEAL team task unit in Iraq during the pivotal battle of Ramadi. After completing his service, Jocko became a business consultant, personal development leader, author, and host of a massively successful podcast.

I had never heard of him until I got a text from my buddy Erik Maier. When it comes to family and friends, I feel like I'm the luckiest guy in the world. Erik has been one of my rocks since we met around 2008. No matter what, I know he is there for me, and I'm there for him.

One Friday that spring, Erik was about to leave work when a new song popped up recommended by Spotify. At first, Erik closed the window on his screen, but for some reason he went back and pressed Play.

The song, "How Dark It Can Get," turned out to be a spoken-word track by Jocko. It was about the similarities between war and cancer. The central refrain of the song goes like this:

> *Now that I know how dark it can get, I truly*
> *appreciate the light in the world.*

Erik is an engineer for a semiconductor company. He's pretty grounded, not generally the type to be looking for signs from God or the universe, so it was even more powerful when he shared the track with me. Nothing like it had ever showed up in his Spotify before.

"This is freaky. I hope it's OK to share this with you," he texted me, with a link to the track. "It might be helpful."

Well, that turned out to be an understatement. Of all the content I have consumed as a cancer patient—books, magazine articles, podcasts, music—the album *The Path* by Jocko and Akira the Don has been the most influential. That album carried me through 2019 and into 2020. I still listen to one or two tracks from it on most days.

Sometimes you get hit by that song or album that's the perfect message at the perfect time. For a guy who was trying to get his swagger back in the face of a shitstorm, Jocko offered up the right medicine.

This is a snippet from one of the tracks, called "Unbroken."

> *There's all kinds of different ways to break. You can*
> *break physically. You can break mentally; you can*
> *break your heart; you can break your spirit; and none*

of these are fun, and all of those are gonna leave a mark. But the mark that they leave can be a mark of victory, or it can be the mark of defeat.

When you break, you have the opportunity to show the world, the whole world, what you are really made of. So if you break, the fight isn't over. In fact, if you break, the fight is just beginning. And as you crawl up and out of that dismal and wretched place, and you're covered in blood and sweat and dirt and filth; as you rise above what you were, and as you take the form of who you are supposed to be, you will see in the very act of standing up, in the very act of fighting on, you will become, and you will remain, unbroken.

Man, I get fired up every time I hear or read those words! That message has become part of my DNA.

Here was Jocko, this diesel truck of a human, this tough-as-nails SEAL commander, someone who had faced death countless times and lost many of his fellow soldiers, telling me that it's OK to be broken—that I can still be redeemed.

It was pure alpha motivation with heart, and that was really the first time another man had given me that kind of guidance. I could glimpse how all of the pain I was going through, physically and emotionally, might eventually become part of my purpose.

Jocko didn't know me, or the impact his work had on me, but I'm forever grateful to him for it.

HOLDING ON

In the United States these days, we are collectively terrified of illness, dying, and death. We're terrified of pain and will do anything, or take any pill, to protect ourselves from it.

With cancer, though, pain is not optional. It's part of the program, and it's going to hurt like hell. Physically and emotionally, you're going to experience pain you could never imagine. There's no getting around it, and there's no skipping past it.

The only thing this pain requires of you is to endure it. Nothing more. Nothing spectacular. In the midst of the pain, you just need to hold on, like a cat hanging from a windowsill. You may not be able to talk or read or even watch a show. You can just breathe and hold on...until you get some more space to function, and eventually thrive.

The upside to all of this pain is that you are fully awake.

As a cancer patient, you are now living a more primal existence, like hunters in days past who faced predators and dangers every day, or workers who constantly face the very real possibility of death.

There will be times when you feel like a warrior, when you will feel the hair stand up on your arms because you are ready to fight for your life, for your family, for the work you need to manifest in this world. Then you will stand and fight.

All that time you once spent thinking about the future, or dwelling on the past, now can be spent living in the present.

All the limitations you imposed on yourself can be lifted. There is no more talk of, "Well, I'll get to that 'someday.'" Someday has arrived.

Any illusions you had about lifespan, expectations of life's milestones, safety, protection from pain—those get burned away with your old self.

STEPPING INTO A NEW LIFE

The positive shift in my cancer journey happened when I stopped trying to get back my old life and stepped into my new one. Most of the time, this new life is bigger, better, more loving, more expansive, more generous, and more disciplined than my life was before cancer. But like I said, the process is hell, and there are no shortcuts.

In 2018, during my first year of cancer, if someone had given me a talk about the silver linings of my disease, I would have stormed away. But by mid-2019, I was ready to accept all the silver linings I could find.

My cancer had recurred, so I'd gone under the knife for a

second liver surgery, again with Dr. Rutstein at Central Maine Medical Center.

Until that point, I had written very little about my cancer experience, which might seem odd to people who know me. I started writing short stories and poetry in elementary school, and then I focused on nonfiction in college. Ultimately, writing became my profession—first as a newspaper journalist and later as a freelance writer and public relations consultant.

At first, I couldn't write about my cancer because of my mental health. But I gradually began writing in spiral notebooks, even when it was emotionally painful, because I knew writing was one of my best tools for processing and understanding my reality.

Four days after my liver surgery in May of 2019, this was my notebook entry:

> *Our youngest daughter plays Little League softball, and today I'm coaching first base. I'm standing just outside the basepath, clapping my hands, looking toward the batter's box where our 11-year-old, Elsie, is about to hit.*
>
> *Up and to my left, in a small wood-framed booth perched over the dugout, my wife Sarah is operating the scoreboard. Our 13-year-old daughter, Sage, cheers on her sister's team. They smile down at me. They are wearing winter hats and coats as it is one of*

those damp, steel-gray afternoons on the coast of Maine. Temperatures in the 40s with full clouds. The kind of day where the batters' bones rattle when they hit the ball, and all we can think about is a sunnier day to come, a 75-degree day in July, when the sun will shine over the Atlantic Ocean less than a five-minute walk from here.

I watch Elsie. I see her look at me, take a big breath, and get into her fierce batting stance. The pitcher rocks backward, springs, and releases the ball. CRACK. A sharp grounder to the shortstop, who scoops up the ball and throws to first for the out.

"Great contact! Way to put it in play!" I smile and pat Elsie on the back as she hustles off.

I shouldn't really be here.

My doctors want me to skip a few games, get some rest, heal from surgery. But I can't help myself. These games, the fun I have with the girls, that's my best therapy. Most of the time when I'm here, I forget I'm a stage IV cancer patient.

Most people at these games don't know about my cancer. They would never guess it by looking at me. They can't see that under my coat and shirt, there is a plastic tube inserted in the left side of my abdomen, allowing blood to drain from my surgical site to a collection bulb in my left pocket.

There is more tubing on my right side, connecting a battery-powered pump to the purple dressing that covers my incision. When I go for my follow-up appointment later this week, my nurse will peel the dressing away and let the wound continue to heal.

There are some people who know my situation. The team members know. They are sweet kids.

"Do you feel good, coach?"

"Yep, I do."

"Did surgery go OK?"

"Yep, thanks for asking."

There are parents who ask as well, mostly the ones who have known me for years. Others just say hello, and there—in that empty space that follows; in the quiet nodding—is the unspoken question.

How long will I live?

It's the only question, really, the one that follows me to every doctor's visit; MRI, CT, and PET scan; blood draw; and all the stuff in between—the softball games, band and chorus concerts, game nights with friends, and walks on the beach with Sarah.

More than a year after my diagnosis, the question doesn't have as much power as it once did. It takes up far less space in the room. It doesn't break me or bring me to tears as much as it used to, and it usually doesn't prevent me from being in the moment and living vibrantly.

But it's there, always around the margins, sometimes quiet, sometimes screaming alarm bells in my nightmares (sleeping or awake).

And if you ask me today for an answer, as I stand here in the aftermath of another surgery, in the gratitude of another softball game, I would tell you the truth as I know it: I don't know.

CHAPTER 6

FINDING YOUR PEOPLE

UNTIL CANCER, I was a social media skeptic.

I enjoyed the ability to share photos and updates easily with faraway friends and family on Facebook, but that was about it. I didn't like the posturing, the popularity contests, and the fakeness of it all. And I really didn't like the political and cultural rage. Social media, I had decided, was largely a cesspool of judgment and virtue signaling.

Having cancer opened my eyes to the highest, most-helpful use of social media—connecting with people who are facing the same life challenges.

Being a 41-year-old stage IV patient, in a rural area, set me apart from most of my peers. We knew of only a couple of people in our small town who had gone through cancer at a relatively young age. The Dempsey Center group was a life-saver, but most of the participants were significantly older than me and most had other types of cancer.

If I had questions about colorectal cancer and its related treatment options and their side effects, or raising children while "cancering," I couldn't just meet up locally with people who were facing the same set of circumstances.

So as I continued on my path toward redemption in 2019, I turned to social media for the connections and knowledge I craved.

I was about to learn the power of the patient-to-patient movement, which helps people like me to not just support one another but to share information that could extend our lives—even save our lives.

The first two groups I learned about were Colontown and the Colon Club. Colontown is a collection of private "neighborhoods" on Facebook, facilitated by colorectal cancer patients, survivors, and caregivers. The Colon Club operates old-school message boards, publishes an annual magazine, and caters to a younger CRC crowd.

I dove in headfirst, reading every post in those places. Just as I felt I had met "my people" at the Dempsey Center, I immediately felt at home when I was in Colontown and the Colon Club.

DR. TOM MARSILJE

When I first found the writings of Dr. Tom Marsilje, through the Colon Club message boards, I didn't even know his name.

I knew him as DK37.

That was the handle Tom used for his posts to online colorectal cancer support forums. Tom was a cancer medicine researcher from San Diego who was diagnosed with stage IV colorectal cancer at age 40. He had two young children, just like me. For five years, between his diagnosis and his death, Tom pursued cures for all of us while spending countless hours helping other CRC patients.

Tom's writings were a treasure trove for patients like me who were seeking hope and reliable information. Tom could provide a primer on the most complex topics, from integrative treatments to obscure clinical trials, using plain language for us non-scientists.

On his blog and through his posts, I learned more from Tom than I did from any other patient or doctor. His posts introduced me to immunotherapy breakthroughs, which would ultimately extend my life.

Tom passed away in November of 2017, shortly before my diagnosis, but the legacy he left in his writings has sustained me, and will do the same for countless more CRC patients well into the future.

More than anything, Tom's writing was kind. It was generous and full of his heart and wry humor. He was honest about our disease, never denying its cruelty and lethality. He was also honest about his hope—his determination to live with joy, diagnosis be damned. Whenever he had the opportunity, he would cannonball into pools, lakes, and ponds. Hell, he probably cannonballed into the bathtub!

At the end of his posts and correspondence, Tom used a

simple signoff to remind us that we can't let the fear of death dampen our passion for living.

To Life. – DK37

———————

COLONTOWN

Tom gave me a direct line to the next magical people in my journey toward becoming a patient leader by pointing me toward the online community Colontown. There I met Erika Hanson Brown, the founder of Colontown; along with Nancy Seybold, Manju George, Steve Schwarze, Todd Mercer, Julie Saliba Clauer, Lindsey Musick, Elaine and Robert Ramirez, and so many other patient leaders and friends in the Colontown community.

Colontown is much more than a support group. It's a virtual think tank where patients exchange experiences and ideas, while moderators keep members informed on the latest scientific developments.

Just over the past few years, Colontown has added learning modules. And some of the world's leading CRC researchers and clinicians give presentations for the membership.

Earlier in my cancer journey I assumed I would learn everything I needed to know about my disease and options from my oncologists, surgeons, and other medical providers.

That wasn't the case.

That is not a knock on my local oncologist. He's a fantastic doctor who has gone above and beyond to connect me with specialists at major cancer centers, including Johns Hopkins, UC San Diego, Dana Farber, and Mass General Hospital.

But even he acknowledges that oncologists are overwhelmed by the number of their cancer patients. They simply do not have the capacity to dig as deep as they would like into each individual case.

They also cannot possibly keep up with the pace of new information emerging from other cancer centers and clinical trials around the world.

Oncologists are also usually focused on their own cancer center and the options they can directly provide. If they don't have an option on hand for you, they usually don't have the capacity to search around the country for options at other centers.

That is where groups like Colontown can bridge the gap.

In Colontown, I can connect with dozens of people with very similar disease biology. I can search a database where patients report their experiences, in real time, on clinical trials around the world. I can ask questions to moderators who have mind-blowing science and medical pedigrees, and they can help me find answers.

"Medical teams care about their patients, but there is no way they can be up on all of the research, clinical trials, and so much more," said Julie Saliba Clauer, a stage IV patient

73

and member of the Colontown leadership group.

"Patients, on the other hand, have a very narrow focus," Julie said. "They are seeking information about treatments and trials specifically relevant to them. Patients can then pass along that knowledge to others with similar cancer profiles."

Since I joined Colontown in 2019 I have not made a single treatment decision without the wisdom and guidance of the community and the friends I've made there.

I quickly moved from just reading posts to contributing my own posts and starting conversations with Colontown members. About a month after I started doing this, I received a private message from Erika, the founder. At first I thought I had violated one of the community rules. Erika assured me that I wasn't in trouble. She'd read some of my posts, and other members had mentioned to her that I might be a potential leader within the community.

Erika was living near Washington, DC, at the time and was visiting Boston for work. She asked if I could come down to Boston to meet her in person; she also invited me to participate in a leadership workshop to be held in San Diego. Not only that, she wanted me to speak at the workshop.

I took about a day to get back to her.

Part of me was ready to step into this opportunity—to become a patient advocate and leader. The other part of me was terrified. All those old doubts crept in, that I wasn't good enough, and that I would let Erika down.... But ultimately the voice of Dr. Tom Marsilje kept echoing in my head. I texted Erika: "I'm in."

After I drove down and picked her up from her hotel, Erika and I drove around the outskirts of Boston. She told me about her own journey as a CRC patient and her vision for Colontown. Then she took me to dinner in Boston, where we met another powerhouse patient advocate, John Novack. He was working for Inspire, which is essentially an online platform for communities based around specific medical conditions. John would become another huge ally for my personal development in the cancer space.

November of 2019 was the month of my coming-out party as a patient leader. It had taken me a year and a half to get to that point, but none of it could have happened any sooner.

I wrote a column for Maine's *Portland Press Herald*, where I had once worked as a news reporter, encouraging people to talk with their doctors about colonoscopies and other screening tools for colorectal cancer.

For the first time since my diagnosis, I posted about my cancer on Facebook.

> So, I guess it's time to start writing about this whole cancer thing. Those close to me know I've been fighting stage IV colon cancer since March of 2018. I've had three surgeries and chemo. As a family, we've been open about this since day one. But today is the first time I'm sharing about it on FB.

My hope is that through writing I can help other patients and families. The first step is a column in today's Portland Press Herald. Thanks for reading!

Then I wrote another column for the *San Diego Union-Tribune*, about my cancer journey, Dr. Marsilje, and the impact of Colontown. Attending Colontown's Empowered Patient Leaders workshop in San Diego in November of 2019 felt like a family reunion.

When I returned to Maine, this was one of the first blog posts I posted to my website.

Finding my people in COLONTOWN: A writer with stage IV colon cancer attends his first patient workshop since diagnosis, and leaves with lifelong bonds

Nov. 18, 2019

What does colorectal cancer look like up close, in person?

It's a proud mother and wife from Kansas City who just went through chemo session #83 and who, come hell or high water, is going to watch her son swim at the Big Ten Championships in February.

It's the kind smiles and tired eyes of a couple from northern California who lost their 37-year-old son to colorectal cancer a year ago and who are stepping up their advocacy work so other parents won't have to endure that grief.

It's a marketing professional who refused to settle for any medical team, so she moved her family from Chicago to L.A., where a world-class oncologist gives her the best shot at making memories with her husband and 2-year-old daughter.

For a weekend when we spend time together, colorectal cancer is a hug we've been waiting for—jokes that make our cheeks hurt from laughter, shared tears, and the wordless longing we all carry. It's the spur-of-the-moment cancer tattoos and scars that criss-cross our bodies like roadmaps.

I'm a writer, husband, and father of two teenage girls. I'm a stage IV colon cancer patient. I'm trusting my instincts and launching into the world of patient advocacy.

I've been encouraged along this path by friends in Colontown, an online information hub and support network for nearly 5,000 colorectal cancer patients and caregivers.

Earlier this month, I had the pleasure of meeting more than 20 of them. We gathered in San Diego for one of Colontown's Empowered Patient Leaders workshops. The idea is for new members like me to learn best practices for helping others within the community and to build on our scientific knowledge of colorectal cancer.

It was the first time since my diagnosis in March 2018 that I was able to socialize in person with a group of people who are facing CRC or have lost loved ones to the disease.

To be honest, I didn't know what to expect in San Diego.

What would my fellow patients be like? Would it be a gloomy weekend?

Not at all.

This was a group of smart, talented, kind, and motivated CRC badasses. Despite many participants being on harsh treatments that assault their bodies and minds, everyone brought energy and innovation to the table.

I quickly realized I was participating in a think tank with the potential not only to change individual lives but to change the delivery of cancer care. This might sound like a stretch to outsiders, but folks in our shoes don't have time for small steps.

Many of the San Diego crew are stage IV patients. Our original colon or rectal cancer has spread to other organs, most commonly the liver and lungs. Many of us are relatively young, in our 30s and 40s, with spouses and kids.

While prognosis varies based on several factors, most patients with metastatic CRC are not alive five years after diagnosis.

All of which makes their participation in the workshop so remarkable. They spend countless volunteer hours online helping other patients and pushing for advancements in science, while knowing that when the next breakthroughs arrive it might be too late to save their own lives.

The model of Colontown is an example of the patient-to-patient movement that is accelerating across all diseases and conditions.

This involves the sharing of information and direct experience related to treatment options, clinical trials, cancer centers, oncologists, surgeons, research, and anything else that might help us—and the patients who follow in our footsteps—get to remission or cure.

I came away from San Diego with clarity and motivation. I also came away with new friends.

One of them is the priceless Manju George, a stage III rectal cancer survivor from Omaha. She is a scientist-researcher and one of the Colontown leaders. We engaged in a brief debate over whether or not CRC patients are brave simply by living with our disease.

She said she didn't think so, because cancer isn't a challenge we asked for.

I looked around the room, estimating the collective surgeries and chemo infusions, CT, MRI, and PET scans. I studied the faces and thought about their stories. I thought about Manju, who spends so much of her time educating others about our disease, encouraging us to advocate for ourselves, and connecting us with the brightest minds in the field of cancer care.

Sorry, Manju, but I'm not backing down on this one.

You are what courage looks like to me.

I had arrived in San Diego as a tentative advocate, dipping my toes into the water, wondering if I had something to offer to the colorectal cancer community and the broader cancer community.

I came home as a patient advocate, ready to change the world.

Thanks to the love and affirmation I received at the workshop, I began posting regularly to my blog, as well as on Facebook, Twitter, and LinkedIn. My messages were resonating with people. I was really beginning to understand how much value we can deliver, patient to patient, online. We can empower patients to be informed, active participants in decisions about their care.

MICHAEL RIEHLE

I want to share with you a couple of personal stories—one patient, and one caregiver—about people who have experienced the impact of the patient-to-patient movement.

Michael Riehle is a guy's guy. He was born and raised in a rural area near Buffalo, NY, hauls vehicles for a living, and proudly wears a thick Viking's beard and a bunch of brightly colored tattoos. He's got a mischievous streak, which I love, and he also has a heart of gold. When I saw Michael posting about his fight with stage IV colorectal cancer, I knew we'd be friends for life.

He was only 31 years old, recently married to his wife, Sara, when he received the shocking diagnosis. At his first cancer center, his medical team didn't give him much hope. He was told to get his affairs in order. He had so much disease in his liver that he was labeled inoperable, incurable.

"I didn't even know what to say. The only treatment offered was chemo for life," Michael recalled. "They told me I probably had a year, maybe more if I was lucky. I started treatment, but my wife and I just could not leave my life in the hands of a team that didn't believe I could live a long, healthy life."

That bleak appointment was on a Friday. Immediately

when they got home, Michael and Sara went online to search for guidance and possibly other options.

They joined Colontown and learned what other patients were doing for similar diagnoses. They even connected with patients who had been told there was nothing that could be done, who had moved on to other cancer centers, and who were now thriving.

"Thankfully, we found Colontown right off the bat," Michael told me. "It led us to a world of information and guidance. With our new knowledge, we got two second opinions and eventually landed at Memorial Sloan Kettering (MSK) Cancer Center NYC. There we met with the team that would completely change the trajectory of my journey."

Michael's team at MSK mapped out a pathway—albeit a narrow one—for him to get to that holy grail of cancer, NED (No Evidence of Disease).

The first step was a colon resection and implantation of an HAI pump, which is a device that delivers heavy-duty chemotherapy directly to the liver. About four months later, surgeons performed the first of two surgeries to remove cancer from Michael's liver. The second surgery took place about three months afterward. He has remained cancer-free for well over a year since his treatment.

"It was exhausting, but it paid off in the long run. It's wild to think that I was given a death sentence more than two years ago, and here I am today with that cherished NED status," Michael said. "I mean, to put it frankly, you have to step up and be able to do some of this stuff on your own, and not rely on your doctors for every piece of information that's out there."

"I have definitely learned the importance of trusting your instincts," he told me. "If it doesn't feel right with your hospital, find one that is the proper fit for you. I am so thankful for these online communities for being such life-changing resources for us. My goal is to bring hope to other cancer patients and show the importance of getting second opinions."

"If I didn't advocate for myself and do my own research and be proactive about my own care, I wouldn't be in the same shoes as I am now," Michael said.

Michael is well aware that his odds of recurrence are high, but he is grateful for every day he lives beyond his original prognosis.

JACQUIE AND RICH EMORY

Jacquie Emory is a force of nature in the universe of colorectal cancer patients.

Originally from Canada, Jacquie was living in Alberta when she met her future husband, Rich, while playing poker on-line. Not long after that Jacquie hopped on a plane for the States, married Rich, and they live in Lilburn, Georgia. She is quick to laugh and quick to cry; she never holds back from telling you how she feels.

If you want to know how tough she is, Jacquie is a regular participant in Spartan Beast races, which are designed to test every aspect of mental and physical strength.

When Rich was diagnosed with stage IV colorectal cancer, Jacquie knew she would need all of her toughness to advocate for his care. The couple received the same initial prognosis as Michael Riehle: Rich would be on "chemo for life," and he wouldn't last long.

"I said, 'No, that's not going to happen,' and probably included a few adjectives in there," Jacquie said. "I went into hyper-protective mode. I refused to acknowledge that this is what his fate would be."

After that bleak appointment with his team, Jacquie went online. She didn't have a medical or science background, but she knew how to connect with people and learn from them. She joined Colontown and lots of its neighborhoods, including Liver Lover's Lane, which is a neighborhood for people like Rich who have disease in the liver. That's where she first learned that some patients were achieving great results from a living-donor liver transplant. Administrator Betsy Post played a key role in helping Jacquie and Rich understand this option.

Dr. Roberto Hernandez-Alejandro, of the University of Rochester, Strong Memorial Hospital, is a leader in living-donor liver transplants for CRC patients. Through the grapevine, Jacquie connected with him.

"We basically fell in love with him as a surgeon," Jacquie told me. "He's a kind, considerate, understanding human being who took our needs into consideration and stood by us through the whole journey."

The next hurdle for Jacquie was to find the right person who would give a portion of his or her liver to Rich. There are no registries for this kind of organ donation, so it usually falls to the patient or their family to find a match. Again, Jacquie turned to social media, making this post.

> What we're about to ask is a life-altering, lifesaving request for Rich Emory's life. We need a living donor for a liver transplant! It is a terrifying and utterly helpless feeling to watch your strong husband fight for life every day. It is also terrifying as we humbly share this in search of a matching living donor to donate a piece of his/her liver to save his life. Fortunately, the liver is a magical organ and will regenerate to just about full size in about three months. We have been granted this chance to save him.
>
> Rich is truly an incredible and genuine man. His love for his son is timeless and his wife immeasurable. He honestly considers so many, including customers at Osteria 832, family and truly cares for them. This is just another aspect of his true-to-life selflessness and generosity as a person. Rich is a gentle soul who saves not only birds, butterflies, and bees, but even snakes and spiders that I'd really rather not see on

my deck! Richard is the most compassionate dad, husband, and friend who we are all proud to have in our lives.

He's not done living! He has adventures not yet realized and a son to watch become the man he was raised to be, and a chance to meet his grandkids. This keeps him fighting every day at the chance of life. Please help us to keep Richard alive!

– Jacquie Emory

One of Jacquie's friends from Canada, David, had done some endurance races with her. When other transplant candidates did not pan out, David stepped up, and he was the perfect match. The transplant surgery was successful, and Rich got a new lease on life.

The aftermath of the surgery was no picnic, with Jacquie struggling to coordinate Rich's post-surgical needs. However, they've gone from zero hope to a new liver and realistic hope.

"It was terrifying to go through that process, but there have to be people to take that chance before it becomes the medical norm," Jacquie said. "So this is us taking the chance, because if we don't, science is never going to advance. We are never going to make progress in colorectal cancer, and we're never going to get a cure."

"Getting the transplant certainly changed the path for both Rich and myself," she said. "And none of it would have happened if we had not advocated for ourselves."

CHAPTER 7

MY GIVING TREE

FROM MY BLOG dated December 20, 2019.

When the storm of cancer hits, you need somewhere to go for protection. Somewhere to shield and strengthen you.

My shield is an oak tree.

It stands alone in the field of tall grasses and wildflowers at the back of our property. Roughly 60 feet tall, with a crown at least that wide, this majestic tree has been a source of strength for generations of Maxwells.

I haven't always protected the tree in return.

A few years ago, vines of American bittersweet climbed up and wrapped around one of the tree's lower limbs. Bittersweet is a menace. It's a creeping vine with twining stems that can grow the length of a telephone pole. The stems wrap around other plants and trees, choking their growth and eventually killing them, unless the bittersweet is cut away.

Under assault, the limb on our oak tree weakened and split. My uncle had to saw the limb off near the trunk.

I walk past the tree every day. Ever since I was diagnosed with stage IV colon cancer in March of 2018, I have made a ritual of walking. After my surgeries, sometimes I'd only walk 50 feet. On my best days, I would walk a few miles, past the oak tree and down the dirt path that leads to the ocean.

In the early months of cancer, those walks were full of resentment.

Intellectually, I understood that life never promised fairness. When you look around the world and see the suffering, this has always been evident. Still, I questioned why cancer had come for me at age 41. Certainly my wife and daughters didn't deserve it.

Walking past the oak tree, I would focus on the sprawling thicket of bittersweet and thorny brambles. The vines were hard at work, wrapping around nearby saplings and the roots of bushes.

The bittersweet was a maddening reflection of the cancer in me.

Lethal. Uninvited. Relentless.

What an awful design by Mother Nature, I thought. I imagined taking a flaming machete and going on the warpath. I wanted to chop and burn every last stem into oblivion. Of course, I knew it would be futile. One has to pick his battles.

So how do we confront our enemies in nature?

For me, I had to start looking at bittersweet and cancer from a different perspective. These are not sentient beings. They don't have thoughts or feelings. They have no intent to kill. They evolve with a singular purpose—to replicate and to survive. This competitive drive is the core design of all living things, whether it's a vine or a cancer cell.

Sure, I can rage against the flaws of our design.

But my quest to be cancer-free doesn't feel right when I'm dwelling in resentment and hate. It feels a lot better when my mission is grounded in my fierce love of my family and friends. There are still plenty of moments when I experience the more destructive emotions. I'm OK with that. I just don't get stuck there anymore.

This shift made it easier for me to see the core lesson offered by threats to our existence—that life is the ultimate privilege.

On my daily walks, I began to focus on the oak tree instead of the brambles.

Yes, the tree was damaged. It had lost a significant part of itself.

And here it stands, undaunted. It continues to weather every gusting wind, every rainstorm, and the deep freeze of Maine winters. Its leaves still return each spring, glorious as ever. It is my giving tree. I spend time with it every day for communion and to offer thanks for its inspiration.

In the tree, I see myself.

I've lost parts. I've been damaged. Yet here I am, standing my ground, living with joy and defiance in the face of the storm.

GAINING CONFIDENCE

When I wrote that post, I had no plans to take that story any further, like making it into a short film.

But all of these helpers—just like Lona, Kate, and others I have shared about—they always seem to emerge at the right time in my life. My friend Roger McCord read that blog post and reached out to me. Roger and I had worked together at the *Portland Press Herald*. Afterward, he moved on to photography and videography. He was one of the first people I knew to use drones.

One morning, I opened up my email and there was a message from him.

Roger McCord here, reporting that I was pretty much gobsmacked by the news of your diagnosis. I see that you have responded with vigor, wit, and courage—leading me to offer some support.

I really like what you've done so far in various media—the oak tree essay was off-scale good, and the bike-riding video clip in San Diego was also very effective.... And yet, there might also be a place in your campaign for a media component that is more structured and, ummm...I dunno the adjective... how about "arty"?

"Hell yeah!" I replied. "I'd love some arty content!"

Roger visited my property three times, his little car jam-packed with cameras and recording equipment. I also visited his studio for some other shots.

The result was a short video that provided a stunning visual companion for my essay. After we shared it on my website and social media, and it made the rounds through Cancerland, I received hundreds of messages thanking us for the video.

I was getting more comfortable and confident about sharing my journey. And I was learning new ways to connect with people in the trenches with me.

My cancer, meanwhile, was stubborn as usual.

By late 2019, I had already undergone a colon surgery, three months of chemotherapy, and two liver surgeries in hopes of achieving long-term remission, or a cure.

Another scan, though, showed the cancer had returned in my liver. There were also scattered cancerous nodules in my abdomen. That's called "peritoneal spread," when cancer crops up in the abdominal cavity. The peritoneum is the membrane that lines that cavity and covers the organs in the abdomen.

Peritoneal spread is extremely hard to treat. When Sarah and I picked up the hard copy of my scan report, reading it in the parking lot, we shared another ugly-crying session. By this point, going to pick up those reports was heaping trauma on top of trauma.

But we did have an ace in the hole, which we had not played yet: Immunotherapy.

GENETIC TESTING AND LYNCH SYNDROME

When I was first diagnosed, back in March of 2018, my first surgeon, the amazing Dr. Sara Mayo at Maine Medical Center, said to me, "You are young for this. I bet you have one of those genetic glitches."

She was right. Genetic testing during my first year of cancer showed that I have Lynch syndrome, an inherited cancer syndrome that increases my risk of developing cancer, potentially at an earlier age than what is typically seen. One of my genes, called PMS2, has a mutation, also known as a variant (a much nicer word). This put me in the higher risk category for cancer, without me ever knowing.

Like I did with the colorectal cancer diagnosis, I spent hours online researching as much as I could understand about Lynch syndrome.

I had the good fortune of connecting early on with Dave and Robin Dubin from New Jersey, the founders of Alive and Kickn. Their foundation's mission is to improve the lives of individuals and families affected by Lynch syndrome and associated cancers through research, education, and screening.

Dave has Lynch syndrome and is a three-time cancer survivor. He loves soccer, hence the "kickn" part of their foundation's name. He has used his passion for soccer as a crossover way to educate thousands of people.

Through the Dubins, my genetic counselor, and other sources, I learned that our individual risk profiles depend on the specific genes affected. Usually, the PMS2 gene is a good variant to have because it does not cause cancer as often as some of the other genes. For reasons that we do not know, I was one of the folks who got hit with cancer.

There were, however, multiple bright spots that came out of my Lynch syndrome diagnosis.

Number one, I let all of my family members know about the diagnosis. At least six of my direct relatives now have the knowledge that they, too, have the syndrome and need to be checked regularly to prevent cancer or catch it early. We are also able to counsel our own daughters. We've already told them the basics and made sure they know that even if they have the syndrome (which is a 50/50 chance for them), that doesn't mean they are going to develop cancer. It just means that they have a higher risk and need to be diligent about screenings.

Number two, having Lynch syndrome made me an excellent candidate for immunotherapy.

IMMUNOTHERAPY

I could spend the next several chapters trying to explain immunotherapy, how it differs from traditional chemotherapy, and the mechanisms behind it, but I actually want you to keep reading, so we are going to skip most of that.

Essentially, immunotherapy is a class of drugs that release the brakes on a person's immune system, allowing it to identify and eradicate cancer cells.

Think of chemotherapy like wildfire. Doctors give us chemo to kill any fast-growing cells in our body, regardless of whether they are cancer cells or healthy cells.

Immunotherapy, on the other hand, is more targeted, and the side effects are usually more tolerable. In the history of modern medicine, immunotherapy is often regarded as the single biggest breakthrough in the treatment of cancer, and it has only emerged within the last 20 years. Checkpoint inhibitors, the bedrock of immunotherapy, were first tested in humans in 2006.

The trouble with colorectal cancer, though, is that most patients do not benefit from immunotherapy. Only about five percent—the patients with highly mutated tumors—are primed to have good responses to currently available immunotherapy.

As it happens, I'm in that five percent.

So when my medical teams saw the spread of my cancer in my abdomen, I received insurance approval and started my new regimen of drugs, Opdivo and Yervoy.

If you are going to take part in a science experiment, why not be on the cutting edge, right?

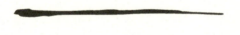

NOT TODAY

I walked with purpose, chest up, shoulders back, into the hallway at New England Cancer Specialists (NECS), ready for my first immunotherapy infusion.

My shirt was plain gray except for two words: "Not Today."

All the nurses and other staff members who watch *Game of Thrones* looked at the shirt and gave me the thumbs up. In the series, the character of Arya Stark, played brilliantly by Maisie Williams, trains in sword fighting.

During their daily lessons, Arya's sword master would always ask the question, "What do we say to the God of Death?"

Arya smiles and answers, "Not today."

If I can borrow some of Arya's badassery, certainly I can pummel this cancer into the forever night.

Before going back to the treatment room, Sarah and I sat down with the nurse practitioner. She walked us through the plan for the infusions, looked over my blood work, and told us about common side effects. She gave us a sheet that listed the bodily systems that can be attacked by an overactive immune system—lungs, intestines, brain, heart, thyroid, adrenal glands, pituitary gland, and skin.

The briefing took about 15 minutes. I signed a waiver giving them consent to treat me and off we went.

There are about 20 reclining chairs in the treatment room at NECS, most of them only separated by a half wall, so you can look around the whole room and also see everything that's going on with your neighbors.

The medication infusion pumps beep constantly. They beep when a drug is close to finishing, when it is finished, when the line is kinked, and when there is an air bubble.

You can always hear the SNAP sound when a nurse clamps a chemo line.

The nurses chat with their patients as they search for the best veins for IVs or insert needles into power ports. Patients ask for pillows, warm blankets, ginger ale, water, coffee....

Most days here, I feel like the youngster. Most of the people in treatment, and the friends or spouses who accompany them, are far older than me. When another "younger" person is getting treatment, we usually make eye contact, and maybe we strike up a conversation. I hate that they are here because of cancer, but it's oddly comforting to have another person in my age bracket getting chemo.

When my immunotherapy drugs come from the pharmacy, my nurse hangs them on the IV pole next to my recliner. She starts my IV and, as usual, I can taste the saline solution as it races through my bloodstream. That's always a good sign: It means the IV line is working exactly as it should.

I put on my headphones and find one of my favorite playlists. The first song is "Regulate" by Warren G because I want to visualize my T-cell army as the regulators, and it is time to mount up.

If I ask myself if there's any fear beneath my bravado, I would have to say yes. But only a touch of fear, an appropriate amount for the situation. By this point in my journey, I can see the fear for what it is—love coming out sideways. I love my life, and I love my family and friends, and I am not ready to leave. That's why I occasionally get a wave of fear, starting in my stomach and rolling up my chest and into my throat.

But those moments are fleeting, with the fear quickly replaced by a peaceful thought, a moment of gratitude—my type of prayer.

After my first two treatments of immunotherapy, I went in for blood work. There is a protein in my blood called CEA (carcinoembryonic antigen), which we use to track the activity of my disease. For some people with colorectal cancer, this blood test is not reliable. For me, it has always been reliable. It goes up when the cancer is growing, and it goes down when it's under control or shrinking.

Lab results are usually posted within a day or two on my patient portal. But the CEA test can sometimes take longer.

I love my patient portal, where all of my lab results, scan results, and other medical records are posted online. However, like many cancer patients I know, I admit to having an unhealthy relationship with my portal. I tell myself, "Trevor, you are NOT going to check obsessively for your CEA result." Then I check obsessively for my CEA result.

It's pretty hard not to do that. I mean, it's only our lives at stake.

We had known for a long time that I might need immunotherapy to control my disease, so this one particular CEA result was pretty crucial.

So I fed the dog, then checked the portal. I folded the laundry, then checked the portal.

Finally, the result was available. My CEA, which had been rising for several months, was falling. The immunotherapy was working! I woke Sarah up because I knew she would want to hear this. I did a little dance at 2 a.m. in our bedroom.

"Not today, cancer," I said. "Not today."

CHAPTER 8

WOLVES

DECEMBER 9TH, 2019, marked my 43rd full turn around the sun.

I walked through the snow and slush with Grace the dog. I worked on my website for this idea I had called Man Up to Cancer. I took Sage and Elsie to rent skis for the winter. We sat down for dinner as a family, then piled onto the couch to watch a holiday baking show.

It was a damn good day.

When you're living with stage IV cancer, especially as a parent of school-age children, you live a jarring double life.

In one, you believe and hope you will live long enough to see your kids graduate from high school, to see them make an impact on the world, perhaps even to meet their children.

In the other, you feel the crushing burden of time. You're frantic to pack in a lifetime of love and memories now, because you don't know when your time will come.

Sage had entered her freshman year in high school. Elsie was in 7th grade. We functioned in that chaotic, high-energy transition between the stuff of youth and the stuff of young adulthood. Gone were My Little Pony and blanket forts. In were *Gilmore Girls* and bedroom doors closed for privacy.

Each day careened toward the next, with the bustle of the girls getting ready for school in the morning going into the bustle of homework, sports, and dinner in the evening.

During that time in late 2019, heading into 2020, Sage sang in her first high school chorus concert. Elsie had her first middle school dance. I set my intention to draw out those moments, to linger in them. Yet when each distinct moment concluded, I was left almost deflated— powerless to slow down time.

In his poem "The Peace of Wild Things" Wendell Berry wisely observes that humans suffer because we tax our lives with forethought of grief.

Our lives would certainly be lighter if we could condition our minds to entirely avoid thinking about our own deaths and how our loved ones will be impacted.

Wouldn't it be helpful if we could let go of tomorrow's troubles? Of course, letting go is easy in the abstract. It's far harder to achieve in real life.

When you love your people so much, and those relationships are under threat, it's hard to avoid the forethought of grief.

My love for Sage and Elsie is beyond words, but I can always try. I love their unique voices, the way they walk, the scrunched-up faces they make when it's too early and too cold to get out of bed on winter mornings. I love the way Sage sways just a bit from side to side when she sings on stage. I love Elsie's laugh when she has her headphones on and she's listening to a book no one else can hear.

I love their warmth, their breath when they hug me, their spirits.

When I'm troubled by the forethought of grief, I try to remind myself that's the natural byproduct of love. I let the grief pass through, and I search out the next moment of connection.

CANCERLAND'S GENDER GAP

At various points during my cancer journey, I would search online for writings, videos, or podcasts about how to be a husband and father while going through cancer treatments and surgeries.

I didn't find much.

There is a glut of content created for cancer patients, but most of it is designed for women or co-ed audiences. Very little content is created specifically with men in mind.

The same gender gap exists in all of the support communities and cancer nonprofits I've encountered. I call it the 3-to-1 Rule.

As much as I love the Dempsey Center and Colontown, women outnumber men in those communities, usually by at least 75 percent to 25 percent. When I would go to group counseling at the Dempsey Center, it was a room full of women, and maybe a couple of guys. Same thing in Colontown. Most of the people participating were women patients and survivors, or women caregivers who were seeking to support their guys.

So many times, I would read posts from wives, daughters, or sisters of men with cancer.

A typical post goes like this: "My husband is stage IV and he is in denial. He doesn't want to learn about his disease or his options. I know he is hurting inside, but he won't open up to anyone. I want to help him, but I don't know what to do."

I often think of a photograph that was taken at an event in Washington, DC, hosted by a colorectal cancer advocacy group. In the photo, about 20 women were gathered around a table, smiling at the camera. In the back left there was one man.

Where are the men? They don't need help facing cancer? Of course they do! They're just too proud, angry, ashamed, or depressed to seek it out.

Research on the gender gap is clear. When facing cancer or another life-threatening illness, men are more likely than women to:

- Withdraw from family and social activities they previously enjoyed.

- Repress emotions and experience embarrassment and shame.
- Practice "solution-based" coping, in which they seek to fix problems independently.
- Struggle with anxiety, depression, and other mental health problems.

These behaviors are cited in research published in journals from the American Society of Clinical Oncology, National Cancer Institute, American Psychological Association, American Cancer Society, and many others.

Researchers at the University of California, Los Angeles (Taylor, et al), put it bluntly in an article published in 2000 by the American Psychological Association.

> *Under conditions of stress, the desire to affiliate with others is substantially more marked among females than among males. In fact, it is one of the most robust gender differences in adult human behavior.*

Men often don't feel comfortable sharing about their cancer in a co-ed environment. In my experience, when men lack communication skills, or when they face a sensitive hardship because of cancer, such as disfigurement or loss of sexual function, they are even less likely to join co-ed groups.

So it shouldn't come as a surprise that the majority of cancer support spaces fail to bring guys with cancer out of their caves.

Michael Riehle, my fellow colorectal cancer patient from up-state New York, agrees. "Men are less likely to seek support because we don't want to be seen as weak," he said. "I know a lot of guys who are loners. They don't think it's manly to express what they are going through, or to be in a position where they feel vulnerable. So when times get tough they can get isolated."

THE HOWLING PLACE

By mid-December of 2019, I was pretty much obsessed with the gender gap in cancer support spaces. I wanted to understand the consequences for male patients and survivors and learn how I might be able to help.

At the same time, I was immersing myself in documentaries about wolves, which I would watch in the middle of the night. My immunotherapy drugs were causing all sorts of inflammation, and the only remedy I had was prednisone, a powerful steroid that kept me up most nights. I had a lot of extra time on my hands.

Wolves are highly intelligent, soulful, and devoted to family. If a wolf is sick or injured, stronger wolves in the pack stay with him and nurture him back to health. If the wolf dies, the others mourn him.

What if men facing cancer had a wolfpack?

105

This, I thought to myself in my prednisone jitters, is going to go one of two ways. Guys are going to love the wolfpack concept, or they're going to laugh and think it's the cheesiest idea of all time.

Here's one of the best things about living the stage IV life: You start to not care about the judgment of others. You don't have time to give a fuck.

You burn your old limitations and you silence those voices in your head that say you aren't capable of doing this—just go back to bed and stop thinking about it. When you get an idea that fires you up, you run after it, sometimes even recklessly.

On one of my sleepless nights, I set up a Facebook group called Man Up to Cancer: The Howling Place. It would be for male patients, survivors, and caregivers of any cancer type, of any age, and in any location.

I wrote down some notes in my journal for an introductory post.

> There are millions of Facebook groups, and probably 2 billion people participating in them. You may be wondering, how is this one going to be different? Here's what I'm thinking....
>
> 1- The Howling Place is where "cancer guys" kick up our feet.
>
> There are many awesome FB groups to learn about

treatment options, clinical trials, medical research, etc., for your specific disease and even your specific tumor biology. For example, I freaking love Colontown and recommend it to all colorectal cancer patients.

Groups like that are where you focus your brain, take care of business, and science the shit out of your illness.

Our group is the laid-back club you go to after business hours. Sure, you can chat about treatments here, but you can also just kick back in a virtual armchair, relax with a whiskey (or soda), and shoot the breeze with awesome guys who totally get you, from all over the world.

We howl about all things cancer. But we also post photos and videos about our families, hobbies, books, sports, travel, cars and bikes, culture, Pomeranians—you get the idea. It's the hangout for "cancer men" that most of us don't have in real life.

2 - Man Up to Cancer outings!

My hope is that we will build on the friendships made here, for get-togethers in real life. I know some of you are already discovering new buddies nearby and making plans to meet. That is awesome!

Down the road, maybe we could plan to meet up

at different locations for group dinners, outings, ball games, etc. I know that's a long-term vision, but when you're a cancer patient there's no time for small thoughts, right?

3 - We are fiercely loyal and ready to take action for our wolves.

Time to get serious. Members of this group and their families are going to need real, actual help.

Many of us will die from cancer. I know we all want to be the ones that make it, but I have to say this out loud. Because if we deny this hard, essential truth, we won't be mentally prepared to help our brothers as they die, and their families after their death.

When a member dies, we will use this group to rally resources. A family might need us to share a fundraising link or to send children letters of condolence and encouragement.

I figured the Howling Place would start small, with a circle of close friends, and would gradually grow as I and others wrote and talked about men, cancer, and isolation.

CAROLINA JOE

The one person I did not anticipate in all my planning was

Joe Bullock, a fellow colorectal cancer survivor. He became a friend who would change the course of my life and the lives of so many others.

While I had been googling "How to be a dad when going through cancer," Joe had been doing the same type of searches. He had experienced the same frustrations when he couldn't find the type of support he was looking for.

"How do I get through this as a dad, as a husband? How do I support my caregiver—my wife—through this as a man?" Joe recalled thinking. "No one was giving me support on how to do this."

Joe is a country boy, born and raised in Durham, NC, where he still lives with his wife Michelle, a nurse at one of the local hospitals. They have two grown children and live on a rural property that abuts a nature preserve.

Cancer has been a theme in Joe's life from an early age. He had a scare with testicular cancer in his 20s. When Joe was in his 40s, his father fell ill with advanced prostate cancer. His father had been abusive to Joe, leading him to leave home as a teenager, but in the final months of his father's life, Joe was the one who acted as a caregiver to him.

Not long after his father's death in May of 2018, Joe himself was diagnosed with stage IIIB colorectal cancer. He had surgery and endured six months of chemotherapy.

He shared his early experience with me.

"When I was diagnosed, most of my male friendships had gone astray. I didn't have very deep relationships in general, especially with men. Because I was a teacher at the time, my work relationships were basically with women," Joe said.

"Women are very good at nurturing, and I felt that support immensely, especially from my wife and daughter," he said. "I felt I just needed more friendships with men who could relate to what it's like to be going through cancer. There were questions, like how to deal with cancer as a man, and how to be the same husband and father in the midst of it all."

"In the beginning, I didn't want to share my thoughts or feelings with anyone. I just wanted to gut through the pain," Joe said. "You just don't show people your weaknesses, and you take care of yourself in this life. That is what my father and grandfather taught me, and that was what I was raised to believe."

But that strategy wasn't working for Joe.

He was depressed, anxious, and felt lost, even months after the doctors had declared him No Evidence of Disease (NED). He was searching for meaning in the aftermath of his treatment.

While I was laying the groundwork for Man Up to Cancer, Joe had been looking for a way to support other men in treatment and survivorship. He was reaching out to other male cancer patients and survivors on Facebook. We didn't know each other well back then, but I would see his posts occasionally in Colontown, and he would see mine.

When I was getting ready to launch the Howling Place, I reached out to Joe to let him know about my ideas.

He was all in.

Joe asked me if he could invite some of his cancer friends.

"Yeah, man, of course," I said, "that's what the group is for."

This is where I underestimated Joe Bullock.

I knew he had been connecting with other "cancer guys," but I didn't know the extent of his network. Within the first week, because of Joe's connections, we had more than 200 members join the Howling Place. We were off and running.

Joe is now the lead administrator of the Howling Place. I lovingly call him the "Cancer Oprah" because he has the biggest heart of anyone I know. He has sent literally thousands of messages, cards, and small gifts to men and kids going through cancer.

I have the privilege of having a close friendship with Joe, collaborating with him, and talking or texting with him every day.

But if Joe ever asks if he can bring a few friends to your party, don't say I didn't warn you.

CHAPTER 9

ROLE MODELS

BY MID-2020, THE Howling Place was thriving. We were reaching men throughout the country and beyond. Some good friends generously offered their time and expertise to help me take the mission to the next level—a Man Up to Cancer podcast.

It was a new outlet for me, drawing on my years as a journalist. It allowed me to connect deeply with other men facing cancer, men who would become lifelong friends. These are people who inspire and motivate me on a daily basis.

Kelin Welborn, a woman artist friend from our small town in Maine, came on as my co-host, providing the much needed perspective of someone outside men in cancerland. Kelin helped me understand the universal themes tied to my experiences as a cancer patient.

For podcast guests, I was looking for male cancer patients, survivors, and caregivers who blend toughness and vulnerability. You might assume that type of man would be hard to come by. But once we started getting numbers rolling into the Howling Place group, I had no trouble finding role models.

Our members were ready to share their experiences with each other and with the world. Some of them had been looking for the right environment—a male-only, judgment-free zone. Once they found it, they didn't need much persuading to connect with one another and break down stereotypes.

The podcast also has been a way for us to show people what it's really like for guys as we experience cancer. All of it. The awfulness, the beauty, and the humor we lean on to get us through.

I'm honored to introduce you to five role models who have joined me as guests on the podcast—Tracy Morgan, Jay Carter, Dave Nitsche, Danny Riggs, and Jared McMillan.

TRACY MORGAN

The first thing about Tracy Morgan is this: Don't let him fool you.

He may come across as a grumpy old Midwesterner, griping about the weather or the news, walking around his town of Grand Ridge, Illinois, population 650.

But give him a few minutes, and you will realize he is the best friend any guy could ever wish for. Tracy is a proud U.S. Navy veteran, a father of three, and a grandfather of 11. He has been living for more than three years with metastatic prostate cancer that spread to his bones in his neck, ribs, lower back, pelvic area, both hips, and right femur.

Tracy is the founder of Mohawk Mission, which calls on men to screen for prostate cancer. He also founded the PC Tribe, an offshoot of Man Up to Cancer's Howling Place where men with prostate cancer can howl.

Before cancer, Tracy kept up the exterior of the "tough guy," the hardass who never needed to see a doctor. He now counsels men on how to avoid that trap.

"Yeah, I was always like, 'I'm fine. Leave me alone. There's nothing wrong with me. I don't like seeing a doctor. It's a waste of my time.' Every excuse you could come up with, I had it. I'm the poster child for stage IV prostate cancer because of that," Tracy said. "Now it's a complete turnaround. My daughters look at me and go, 'Where's dad at? Where is that quiet guy who never used to say anything? We can't shut him up now!'"

"I was pretty open, after the first couple weeks of the 'Why me?' stuff that you go through, and I finally accepted it. Okay, I got it. What am I gonna do about it? I'm sure God is sitting there saying, 'Well, you have this now. What are you gonna do with it?' I'm like, 'Well, I guess I'd better help some people with this. I got the opportunity to do it. Let's do it.'"

JAY CARTER

Jay Carter is a true renaissance man. A native Californian who now lives in Dallas, Jay has a wide array of skills in software engineering, graphic design, marketing, social media, music, and more.

Two things made me gravitate toward Jay when I met him online, where he goes by the handle @thatcancerdude. First, his smile fills up a whole room. Second, he is an outdoor-adventure fanatic—snowboarding, paddle boarding, skiing, white-water rafting. All of the outdoor-adventure photos and videos I saw of Jay were taken after his recovery from intense chemotherapy and a life-saving stem cell transplant in 2012–13.

Jay is now in his late 30s, but he was diagnosed at age 26 with chronic myeloid leukemia (CML). During his extended period of treatment, Jay's father was facing prostate cancer while his grandmother was facing breast cancer.

Before cancer, Jay had graduated from the University of California at Davis and was on track to train in the medical field. He was considering physical therapy or orthopedic surgery. He moved to Dallas from Sacramento in part because he landed an internship at a Dallas hospital, and also to help care for his father. Three months later, Jay was diagnosed with CML.

In recent years, Jay has been involved as a participant, volunteer, and consultant for organizations that provide support for cancer patients, including Epic Experience and Reel Recovery.

"What's one thing you know now, but wish you had learned earlier in the journey?" I asked Jay before our podcast conversation.

"The journey never ends. Life doesn't miraculously return to normal once treatment is complete and remission is obtained," Jay said.

"There will be good days—enjoy those. Other days will not be as pleasant. Take time in those moments for yourself, while being mindful of the fact that just like the good days the bad days will not last forever. No matter what comes your way, you will be alright. Your mind is a powerful tool. Put it to use in your favor."

———————

DAVE NITSCHE

Dave Nitsche of Calgary, Alberta, Canada, has every reason to be bitter.

His cancer diagnosis came at age 50, when Dave began having vision problems in his left eye. The problems got so bad that doctors had to remove his eye. When the tissue was tested in the lab it revealed cancer, which had spread from his lungs. An oncologist basically told Dave that he was going to die, and it would probably be soon.

Dave wasn't going to accept that, so he got the best care possible, learned all he could about his options, and connected with others walking a similar path. He has been on two targeted therapies that have kept his disease stable. And he has resumed one of his great passions, hiking with his dog Indie in the scenic wilderness of Western Canada.

He also speaks up as an advocate for lung cancer awareness as well as advances in research and treatment.

Dave has always been able to rely on his body and mind working in sync. He is accustomed to pushing both to the extreme as an ultra runner and Ironman athlete. Starting when he was a Winnipeg native up until his diagnosis, he had trained for literally thousands of hours over the course of decades. He then applied many of the lessons he learned during training to his cancer journey.

"In the sense of the long triathlons, everything changes," Dave said. "You can be in the middle of the swim and around 2000, and you're getting bashed around, and things are looking shitty. You're having a panic attack—can't breathe—and you're swallowing water up your nose. And then all of a sudden you find open water...and you start getting into your rhythm."

"And you're feeling good, and then you get on the bike and, well, you get a flat tire," he said. "Well, what are you gonna do? You're not gonna stop; you're not gonna quit. You change the tire, and you keep going. So, you know, there are parallels to that in cancer."

DANNY RIGGS

"I'm that 1 in 833."

Those are the words of my friend Danny Riggs of Houston, Texas. Roughly 1 in 833 men will be diagnosed with breast cancer in their lifetimes. They face the confusion, stigma, and additional isolation of coping with what is primarily a women's cancer.

Yes, men get breast cancer. If you have a lump, pain, swelling, or anything unusual going on with your breasts or nipples, talk to your doctor.

Danny is the proud husband of Sarah, and the father of two sons and a daughter. He has had multiple careers: he started out as a paramedic but most recently worked as a safety manager and supervisor in the construction industry.

Danny is also one of the Howling Place's 18 Wolfpack leaders from across the U.S. and Canada. In that role, he talks to other people in the cancer community about the Man Up to Cancer mission and helps connect them to resources like the Howling Place.

Along with Michael Riehle from South Wales, NY, and Don Helgeson from Nanaimo, BC, Canada, Danny planned and executed the first annual in-person retreat for the Man Up to Cancer community. It was called the Gathering of Wolves and it was held at Camp Duffield in Delevan, NY, in the fall of 2022.

In my podcast episode with him, Danny, in his typical no-holds-barred fashion, talked about what it was like to get the diagnosis, to endure the treatment, and to navigate survivorship.

"A lone wolf will not survive," Danny said. "I have been a lone wolf in a lot of things that I've done in my life, especially when I say I'm the provider, I'm the fixer, I make it happen. And then when I got diagnosed, I wasn't able to do that anymore. When I was going through treatment, I couldn't do that anymore."

"If you don't ask for help, nobody knows you need it," he said. "The power of the Howling Place group, the transparency and honesty, it's been such a blessing to be part of it. It's a 'pay it forward' type of thing. And the best part about it is that I'm never going to be done paying it forward, because I have realized that the more I pay it forward, the more I get out of it. I feel better by doing more for others."

JARED MCMILLAN

In our group, Jared McMillan was known as Ironwolf.

He earned that nickname because he traveled one of the hardest roads imaginable, with multiple brain surgeries, abdominal surgeries, radiation burns, and metastases throughout his body; and because he loved pumping iron in the gym.

Jared was an Air Force officer who was forced to retire in his 30s to instead fight stage IV colorectal cancer. His favorite hashtag was #FaithFamilyFight. He and his wife Christy welcomed their daughter to the world shortly after Jared was diagnosed. He lived with cancer for five years before passing away in March of 2021.

Words cannot begin to capture the impact that Jared had during his 38 years on earth. All of us in the Man Up to Cancer community admired Jared for his resilience, courage, strength, leadership, and big heart. Jared did not lose the battle. He WON by the way he lived his life.

When I had Jared on the podcast, I asked him about sharing his emotions.

"With all the motivation and inspiration, because that is definitely at the core of who you are, you also have been honest about the darker emotions—fear, sadness, anger," I said. "So rather than pushing those feelings away, or denying they even exist, you have shared about those as well. Why was that important for you? And did that take time?"

"It did take time. Ever since I took on more of a leadership position in the military, I didn't particularly like showing that I had weakness, because I didn't want my troops or anybody else to see that side of me," Jared said.

"Basically all that stuff had been building and building, and I talked to Christy as much as I could," he said. "You know, sometimes I wear a false mask of happiness.... And finally, one day, I just started crying, and didn't stop for two hours. Christy essentially talked me into getting in with a therapist, and talking with them, and seeing what they could help me with. I'm glad I did."

ANNIVERSARY

I wish I could introduce you to so many more of my friends. I will just say that the quality of the men who have joined the Man Up to Cancer community is above and beyond anything I could have imagined.

They are role models in every sense of the word.

On December 31, 2020, one year after I opened the doors to the Howling Place, I posted a thank you to the members.

CALLING ALL WOLVES

Happy anniversary!

One year ago, around 5 a.m., I nervously clicked the button to launch the Howling Place group.

That was after three nights of insomnia, jacked up on prednisone, learning about wolves and pack life. This group is built upon a simple yet powerful concept—that men don't need to face cancer on their own; that we are better off going through it as brothers.

The idea of men supporting other men is not new. It is ancient. But in many cultures, including here in the US, we've been robbed of that heritage. We've been told that we can handle everything on our own, and that we are weak if we accept help. Frankly, that's bullshit.

When I learned to accept help, about six months into my cancer journey, I gained strength I never knew I possessed. I also became better at offering help to others, which is something I have not always been good at.

I'm so grateful to call you all brothers. Joe Bullock was on board from day one, and he stepped up to lead the administration of our rag-tag crew. He reached out and invited most of you to join us. With his endless acts of kindness, he sets the tone for how to treat one another. Joe, you already know how I feel about you, but I'll say it again: You're a hero.

Others—you know who you are—have also taken a big leap of faith to share your hearts and souls with all of us in this forum. It also takes effort to make a group special. The effort here has been truly inspiring.

In this group over the past year you have lifted each other up in the toughest of times. You have celebrated with each other the good news, the milestones, the small joyous moments, the stuff of lives well lived.

You have given each other guidance and information that has changed lives for the better, not just for members but for our families and friends.

You have mourned with each other as our members have died, and you have made the solemn commitment to pick up their banners and carry them forward.

And during a shit year in so many ways, you have brought some light into the darkness.

With all my heart, thank you for being here.

CHAPTER 10

CHEMO ZOMBIE

Sometimes the best map will not guide you.
You can't see what's round the bend.
Sometimes the road leads through dark places.
Sometimes the darkness is your friend.

– Bruce Cockburn, "Pacing the Cage"

ANGER HAS BEEN one of the trickiest emotions for me during the cancer journey, along with its companions, bitterness and resentment.

I don't think I have examined my anger nearly enough. I don't think I've given it enough space to breathe, or the proper outlets to get it out. That's probably because I'm someone who is concerned about how my emotions affect others. No emotion affects others more, or is more unsettling, than anger.

Also, if you're a cancer patient expressing anger, you run the risk of being judged as ungrateful. We know cancer muggles (people who have never faced a cancer diagnosis) prefer it when we, the patients, exhibit positivity, perseverance, and gratitude at all times. To do otherwise would be discouraging to them. And obviously it's our job to comfort the muggles while we are clinging by our fingertips to the windowsill of life. Eye roll.

No matter how much you stuff it down or keep it hidden, anger is a normal human emotion when living with cancer: It's going to find a way to come out.

Sometimes, when I see some 80-year-old dude ripping into an entire pack of Marlboro Reds, eating fast food, and topping it all off with a few vodka nips, I get angry. Why did I get cancer at 41 while this guy just keeps on rolling for decades while checking off every box for poor health?

I know that's unfair, but I have to be honest. I get pissed off on occasion.

I've heard plenty of other patients say, "I don't have the right to get angry." "Look at this other person, or that person—they have it worse." "It would be worse to be a child." "It would be worse to be a parent."

And I totally get that and 100 percent agree in theory.

The problem with that approach, in my opinion, is that it often suppresses anger—a real, valid, powerful emotion that needs to be processed.

Because no matter your circumstances, there is grief that accompanies a life-threatening illness. It impacts your life and the lives of those close to you, and that grief sometimes manifests as real, put-your-fist-through-the-drywall anger.

Your pain is your pain. Your fear is your fear. Your grief is your grief. That doesn't change because you look at someone else's pain and say, "That's worse than what I'm going through."

SOUTHWEST'S BOARDING LINE

In early 2021, on a trip to visit my father and his fiancée in Davis, California, my anger came out sideways.

It was a bucket-list trip because my cancer was progressing. We had never been to California as a family: We wanted to see the Pacific Ocean, the redwoods, and some cities together because we didn't know if we would ever get the opportunity again.

For background, we have never been frequent flyers, other than an occasional vacation or for my trips to cancer centers for second opinions. Our itinerary for our California trip went like this: Fly Southwest Airlines from Portland, Maine, to Baltimore; then fly from Baltimore to Las Vegas; and finally fly from Las Vegas to Sacramento.

Southwest has a confusing ticketing process, at least for those of us who don't travel much. They don't have assigned seats, so basically, once you get on the plane you can take any open seat.

But when you're boarding you're supposed to line up according to your assigned group, based on the time you checked in online. The four of us—me, Sarah, Sage, and Elsie—wanted to make sure we could sit together so we checked in online as early as we could.

At the airport in Baltimore, when it's time to board for our connection to Las Vegas, the gate agent tells everyone to get in their designated boarding groups.

Well, a bunch of young guys who (we later found out) are supposed to be behind us in the boarding line rush forward in front of our family and basically take our spots. They're going to Las Vegas to party, and they're already rowdy.

Nothing sets me off quite like entitlement. So I take our family up to the front of the line, where we're supposed to be, and I try to cut in. I show the rowdy guys our tickets.

One of the guys, probably in his late 20s, gives me an arrogant, disgusted look.

"It's open seating, bro. Get to the back of the line," he says.

I feel the heat rise up through my chest, just like it did at Panera in 2018.

"No. We're not doing that. This is our spot. That's how it works," I say, still at a simmer.

He raises the stakes.

"Dude, it's just a line. We got here first."

127

My simmer is reaching a boil. Sarah's watching me and knows the shit is about to hit the fan. The girls are looking at us, wide eyed. I think to myself, "I'm going to crush this guy, end up in a federal detainment facility, and there will be no California trip." I want to bring down the heat, but it isn't working.

There's no way in hell I'm taking my family to the back of the line. No chance. We have gone through too much to put up with this kid's shit. At some point, even in an airport, you've got to stand up for yourself and the people you love. Meanwhile, the guy continues to run his mouth at me.

I gather my family in my right arm, pulling us together in a circle in front of my nemesis, forcing him back. I turn around and stare him down with all the fury of my cancer hell.

"Yeah, I'm right here, bro," he says. Mind you, this guy is not big. I tower over him, and if I let myself, I could pummel him into oblivion.

But I have already proven my point. We stand our ground ahead of him and his group in line. I ignore his chirping as we get on the plane....

And then we go enjoy the hell out of our vacation.

As I reflected on that confrontation, I knew it wasn't really about our places in that boarding line.

I'm sure that guy has his own burdens to carry, but he probably has no idea what real hardship is.

His first thought each morning probably isn't, "How do I survive this disease that's trying to kill me?"

Of course he didn't know my cancer was the reason our family was going to California (in the midst of my never-ending treatments).

He had no idea that after California I would fly directly to Baltimore, so doctors at Johns Hopkins could maneuver a scope down my throat and poke holes through my stomach so they could take biopsy samples of the tumor that's been growing in my abdomen.

And that's not his fault. I'm glad he doesn't have to understand those realities.

I wouldn't wish cancer on him.

But in that moment, in Southwest's boarding line, he embodied all of the people who cannot even begin to understand my pain and the pain of millions of others like me. I wasn't angry because some guy was a jerk. That happens all the time. I was angry because my cancer won't go away; I'm still fighting for my life; and that's really freaking hard for my family.

A CLINICAL TRIAL

Immunotherapy had kept my cancer stable for much of 2020.

By the early part of 2021, though, several tumors in my abdomen had started to grow. One of them, the big one I called my "problem child," was growing fast and filling up the space between my stomach and liver.

Along with its growth came increased nausea, discomfort, and lack of appetite.

I was at the three-year mark in my journey and, as usual, the hardest part for me was seeing the emotional toll on my family. The girls were still doing great in school, despite the coronavirus pandemic and the ongoing pressure of having a parent with metastatic cancer. Sarah was still her stellar self at her work, carrying the burden of our family's income and insurance.

I could see their stress, the longing for freedom from my illness. With each MRI or CT scan, I desperately wanted to say to them, "I'm all clear. There's nothing to be concerned about now." Instead, most of my scan results brought us all pain.

"Just a setback," I would say. "I'm going to just keep doing what I'm doing. I have great doctors, great care, and we just need to keep living and pushing forward."

But a lot of times, there's nothing to do except cry it out. Sometimes it's a mess, even when we're all doing everything we can to love one another and to "be OK." That can be a helpless feeling, and one that's hard to describe.

I try to always remind people of the impact cancer has on our caregivers. Sarah and the girls have been so brave and incredibly loving. They also each carry a burden that people can't see by looking at them. When you see them at the grocery store, the park, or the town hall, they may look like every other wife or daughter. Meanwhile, they're holding up the whole world inside themselves.

My next move was a clinical trial at The Sidney Kimmel Comprehensive Cancer Center at Johns Hopkins Hospital in Baltimore. The regimen was a combination of two immuno-therapy drugs—Opdivo, which I had already been taking, plus Relatlimab, a newer drug that targeted a different immune pathway. I flew to Baltimore each month for treatment.

There's a common misperception about clinical trials. Most people think trials are "Hail Mary" attempts to turn things around when the cancer has gotten so bad there are no other options. That's absolutely not the case.

The truth is, if you have advanced cancer and are near the end of life most clinical trials will NOT enroll you. Participants must be healthy and strong enough to qualify. Clinical trials for cancer often combine standard-of-care therapies with new drugs. Those combinations sometimes give patients their best chance possible for long-term survival. It's like getting access to the next generation of treatments.

A mistake I see a lot is that patients don't consider trials early enough in the journey.

Unfortunately, in my case, the clinical trial didn't work. My "problem child" tumor grew to 12 cm, and I needed a new plan.

KITCHEN SINK CHEMO

It was time to bring out the big guns—"kitchen sink chemotherapy" (where they throw everything at the cancer at one time). We needed to go big because if we couldn't control the rapidly growing tumors in my abdomen things could go downhill pretty fast.

The hope was that chemotherapy would shrink my tumors so that I might be eligible for surgery later in 2021 to remove anything that remained after we nuked it with chemical warfare.

Kitchen sink chemo for me was Folfoxiri plus Avastin. It was a potently toxic brew of folinic acid, fluorouracil (5FU), oxaliplatin, and irinotecan. I already knew a handful of other colorectal cancer patients who had been on this combination. Basically, they told me to buckle up for all the side effects—nausea, vomiting, diarrhea, sweats, brain fog, nerve damage, nosebleeds, fatigue, throat spasms, hair thinning, cramps, and dizziness.

Bring it on!

After my first infusion, I posted the following on Facebook.

1- A week ago I got my mediport reinstalled so I can receive chemo through a central vein. I had a port when I did chemo three years ago but took it out. Been using my arms and hands for all my IVs. Long story for another day.

2- Had my first FOLFOXIRI chemo treatment on Thursday.

3- Had to miss Sage's track meet Saturday because I was getting my chemo pump disconnected. Boo.

4- Spent Sunday with Sarah and Sage watching Elsie play softball.

5- Not really sure what happened Monday through Wednesday. #chemofog

6- Feeling more human today. Enjoying the porch swing. Thankful for my family and friends. Tomorrow? Who knows! I might surprise you!!

For my second infusion, I made another post. At this point in my journey I had more than 4,000 friends on Facebook. Nearly all of them were patients, survivors, caregivers, or other people touched by cancer. With my posts, I always wanted to keep things real and show my solidarity with them.

Back in the chair for chemo day!

Another shout out to the cancer thrivers....

133

To those of you living scan to scan, infusion to infusion, surgery to surgery.

To those of you losing hair, losing parts of yourself, losing precious time.

To those of you digging deep to attend the ballgames, recitals, graduations.

To those of you who feel like you're trapped inside the glass, looking at the world outside pass you by.

You may feel lost. You may feel scared. You may feel broken.

But let me assure you. You are not alone.

Here, inside the glass, there are millions of us to hold you up.

We know you can do hard things—things you never imagined you could do.

Because while your body may feel weak, your spirit remains invincible.

My friends were right about the side effects of kitchen sink chemo. It was hideous. I was on a two-week schedule. I would go for chemo on a Friday, then take a chemo pump home for the weekend so it could deliver 5FU for 46 hours. Then I would go back to the cancer center for pump disconnect on Monday.

As the infusions went on, I found myself feeling less and

less human. I might only get a few days of feeling somewhat normal during each cycle. I recorded a podcast episode called "Chemo Zombie."

The day before chemo, I would be enjoying life with my family. Then I would go for chemo and I'd turn into a zombie.

I would become disengaged, sick to the very core of my being, drowning in that toxic chemical soup. I would be nonverbal, slumped in the bed or on the couch. When I did get up I would stumble around.

I was there, but I wasn't there.

Sarah and I would actually say goodbye to each other before each session: "See you in about a week."

The real effects of chemo are rarely shown in popular culture. Once in a while you'll see a movie or TV show where someone—usually a woman—is undergoing treatment. It's all very maudlin and overacted. Except for being bald, the woman usually looks WAY too good for actually being chemo sick, because, well, the full truth of chemo doesn't really appeal to audiences.

After my chemo treatments, I knew what I was supposed to do: Hydrate; keep moving; and eat good, nutritious food. I know some people are able to do those things.

For me, the first several days after Folfoxiri, I just held on for dear life. I learned to go back two or three times to the cancer center for IV fluids because there was no way I could keep up with drinking enough fluids at home.

My medical team gave me four different prescriptions to alleviate my nausea, but, honestly, the medicine that helped me the most was cannabis. Whoever came up with the Purple Punch strain of THC, thank you. Using my vape pen was sometimes the one thing that could settle down my nervous system and interrupt the nausea.

I had zero appetite, and when I could eat, everything tasted like cardboard dipped in metal. Sharp flavors sometimes cut through, so I would go to mustard, pickles, and spices. In those first several days after pump disconnect, taking a shower would feel like an Olympic victory. My blood pressure was so low that when I stood up, no matter how slowly, my eyes would go black for several seconds.

Chemo messes with my brain. When I'm incapacitated in bed, dark thoughts creep into my mind. I tell myself I can't do this anymore. I have to remind myself that it's the toxic chemicals at work.

Now that I have terrified you with the reality of my chemo experience, I need you to hear this: Every chemo experience is different. The side effects that hit me might hit you to a lesser extent, or not at all. Some of the guys I know had minimal nausea, even through the most aggressive chemo. Some were able to work and exercise and maintain a more normal routine.

If you are on chemo now, or about to start it, you can absolutely get through it. It demands so much of us, but we are fully equipped to endure it.

There are some lessons that can only be learned in the dark. I put sticky notes on my bedside table to remind me. One is a quote that my grandmother would say to us.

This too shall pass.

Another sticky note reminds me that while my brain cycles through fears and doubts, questioning if I'll ever feel better, I can trust that underneath the anguish my fighting spirit remains whole.

You are not your thoughts.

The last one is our rallying cry and the number-one hashtag in the Howling Place.

#KFG. Keep Fucking Going.

JASON RANDALL

Jason Randall is a stage IV colorectal cancer warrior, Navy veteran, and family man from Eudora, Kansas. He lives with his wife, Tellena, and their three children. He has become a fierce patient advocate and a source of inspiration and knowledge for other patients and their families.

Jason has been through a lot of chemotherapy during the five years since his diagnosis. He has also endured seven surgeries, Y90 radiotherapies, fistulas, a perforated bowel, biopsies, chemical burns, and the loss of more than 100 pounds. In short, he is a cancer badass.

He is a leader in Colontown and is also a leader and administrator in the Man Up to Cancer community.

In 2021, I had Jason on my podcast to share his top five tips for making chemo suck less. No matter which regimen, or the type of cancer you have, these tips are timeless.

Integrative Medicine

Think of integrative medicine as complementary to standard of care (accepted mainstream practices), not as an alternative. It basically entails diet, mental health tools, side-effects control, and high quality supplements that don't interfere with your standard treatments. It's more of a holistic approach. A lot of times oncologists will disregard it so you may have to push for these things. I was in a unique situation because I met my integrative medicine doctor at my NCI center, the same center where my medical oncologist worked, so they were able to speak directly.

Music Therapy

I have daily routines. I wake up and listen to certain music (reggae has always been a big one for me, ever since high school). I've done music therapy where I take lyrics of songs, no matter what they deal with, and relate them to my cancer experience. It's almost spiritual in a way to connect to the words.

I'll just sit there and crank it to like 65 and just let every beat hit me. I may sound crazy explaining this, but it works."

Meditation
I do a very specific meditation called psychosomatic wellness based on the work of the doctor Candace Pert, who is deceased now. The majority of her work is based on neuroscience, music, and the mind-body connection.

One day this specific meditation clicked for me. I don't know where the heck I went, but it was very healing. You know, some people may call it healing energy; some people call it God; and some people call it universal energy. Whatever it is, I connected with it, and it lifted a lot off my shoulders. My advice is to stick with meditation. Don't give up on it—find ways to make it work for you.

Family
I have a very supportive family, including extended family. I know not everyone has that luxury. But if you do, your core family is crucial. If there is someone toxic within your extended family circle, avoid them, that's all I can say. It's hard, and there's no easy way to do it, but you've got to do it for yourself. Remember: Family can be created as well; it's not necessarily just who you're related to.

Movement

There are certain situations where you just can't move, so don't beat yourself up about that. But once you feel motivated to move, don't let that feeling go—get up and move! It sounds so simple, but it's so true. You have to keep moving. I have a very specific playlist, a set of songs I play; when I listen to that I'm walking around like I own the place.

With these last four cycles for me, on that very first cycle, I was out five days straight. I had to take off work. I slept about 15 hours for each of two of those days. And then for the last three cycles, I haven't had a single down day; it was all because I just got up and moved.

– Jason Randall

CHAPTER 11

A MAN'S ROADMAP FOR LIVING WITH CANCER

TO LIVE WELL during cancer, and to give yourself the best chance at survival, you cannot and must not be passive.

You must get assertive about your treatment, your mental health, and your quality of life. You must be the squeaky wheel. Ask questions. Demand explanations. Learn about your disease. Challenge your insurance company, or anyone else who stands in the way between you and your cancer-free future.

I think of myself as the chief executive officer, the CEO, of my cancer journey. My lead oncologist is the chief operating officer, and all the other providers and helpers are consultants that we work with to carry out our mission—keeping me alive.

Because this is the cold, hard truth: No one cares about your life as much as you.

The medical–industrial complex is not designed to go the extra mile for you. In fact, it is designed to spend as little time and effort on you as possible. The system is built

141

to process millions of patients and, frankly, to maximize profit. Many oncologists work on 15-minute appointment schedules, and waiting rooms look like lines at a grocery deli counter. The system is built on efficiency for processing the masses.

Doctors simply do not have the capacity to make YOUR case their most important case. And they don't have all the answers.

I'm not being harsh on our medical providers. Many of them are outstanding, and we love them. But even if you have the smartest, most compassionate team, they are still overwhelmed trying to keep up with all the people who need care.

I'm not telling you to be a jerk. Don't be rude or disrespectful. That works against you every time, and it's bad karma.

But you have every right to be assertive, and it might just save your life.

With all of that said, please remember that none of us has this figured out. There is no "best way" to go through cancer, and you should be wary of anyone who promises you a singular path, especially if it seems too good to be true.

I share the following suggestions because I've been in the trenches for a while, and I've learned some lessons that have helped me. When I started on this road nearly five years ago, I didn't know anything about cancer or how to cope with it. It has been messy and chaotic, and I have so much that I still don't know or understand.

As patients, we are forced to meet each situation and make decisions in real time, in the context of everything else going on in our lives, and often with limited resources.

Be kind to yourself. Trust that you will forge the only authentic road possible for you.

Before I walk you through my four most important tips, the ones that have helped me live well with cancer, let me tell you what they are.

- Get a second opinion.
- Open the toolbox for mental health.
- Take part in the patient-to-patient movement.
- Play.

GET A SECOND OPINION

A few years back, I met a fellow stage IV cancer patient online. Jim was a stone mason from Florida who had worked all the way up from being a helper, to an apprentice, to owning his own business with a crew of five employees.

Jim was rightfully proud of his achievements. He was accustomed to solving his own problems and never asking for help.

After ignoring symptoms for more than a year, including coughing up blood and experiencing short-term memory problems, Jim finally went to see a doctor. Jim went through a battery of tests and scans and was diagnosed with lung cancer that had spread to his brain. He went to see a local oncologist, someone who was a friend of his brother. Jim was put on chemotherapy and was given six months to a year to live.

I asked Jim if he had gotten a second opinion.

"Why would I get a second opinion?" he asked me. "This guy is a good doctor. He is someone my family trusts. If there was something out there that could help me, I'm sure he would know about it."

Jim was also concerned about hurting his doctor's feelings. He felt that if he asked for a second opinion, that would be a show of distrust.

Sadly, Jim passed away before I could speak with him again. I did, however, get a chance to review some medical notes from his case. Jim's oncologist never ordered any tests to see if he would have been a candidate for targeted therapies or immunotherapy. There was a note saying that Jim's wife had asked about seeking a second opinion, but that never happened.

Jim's attitude reflected that of many men I've met over the past five years. They believe all oncologists and surgeons have the same knowledge and skills. They also don't want to offend their doctors.

I understand where these men are coming from, but those beliefs are outdated, wrong, and sometimes even deadly.

Second opinions are absolutely crucial to your goal of survival.

Even the best doctors and cancer centers in the world sometimes miss things on a scan, miscommunicate results, or make mistakes. I had two hospitals (including a highly rated cancer center) tell me that a lesion on my liver was benign. Three months after those opinions, we found out it was cancer.

Individual doctors do not know everything about your cancer or the advances happening around the world that might relate to your treatment.

Global advances in oncology—including the rapid pace of drug development and the mind boggling number of clinical trials—cannot possibly be tracked and absorbed by one doctor or even one institution. In the old days, that might have been possible. But in today's world, the treatment of cancer is collaborative.

The best oncologists and surgical oncologists embrace your request for second opinions. They are not challenged or offended by it. They know second opinions are helpful and necessary, and they will help you overcome logistical hurdles. Your oncologist and your primary care physicians should be ready to go to bat for you if insurance gives you a hard time.

If your doctor or medical team resists your request for a second opinion, that is a huge red flag. You should consider finding a forward-thinking doctor.

Jason Randall, my stage IV CRC brother from Kansas, is one of the most proactive patients I have ever met. By learning about his disease, and speaking with multiple practitioners across a wide range of oncological disciplines, he has made himself the CEO of his journey.

Jason had so much cancer in his liver that the odds were super low that he would ever reach the point where he would be eligible for surgery.

Yet Jason's research, and talks with many other patients, led him to Dr. Yuman Fong, a cancer surgeon at City of Hope National Medical Center in Duarte, California. Jason had to convince his local medical team that the surgical route was possible. They were skeptical, but they ultimately supported Fong's plan.

"For about a year and a half, I was told I would never have a surgery. I'd never be operable," Jason said. "And then I got that second opinion, and it changed everything. I went through a massive surgery. Now my prognosis is totally different than it was. I'm no longer looking at indefinite chemo."

So to finish this section, imagine me raising my voice a bit.

I don't care if you have the highest rated oncologist on the planet. Get a second opinion!

OPEN THE TOOLBOX FOR
MENTAL HEALTH

Ever since November of 2019, when I started sharing publicly about my cancer journey, I have been open about my struggles with anxiety, depression, and the mental health burden of cancer.

I talk a lot about my counselor, Patti, and how my sessions with her essentially saved my life, empowering me to become a patient advocate. I also talk a lot about my experience with group counseling.

For me, as a verbal processor and someone who does not mind sharing my feelings in most types of settings, counseling continues to be a powerful tool. It might be for you as well.

But it's not for everyone. For some guys, the terms "counseling" or "therapy" send them running for the hills. Many of the guys in the Man Up to Cancer community recoil at the idea of sitting around and sharing their feelings.

And that is perfectly OK.

There are also barriers to accessing a qualified mental health counselor, including waitlists, insurance limitations, and financial barriers. There are new apps and digital platforms designed to help patients with our mental health concerns, but the quality of care is inconsistent.

Fortunately, traditional counseling is only one tool in the mental-health toolbox. What matters is that you acknowledge your mental health struggles and then find the right tools to match your personal coping style.

- Move your body, exercise, and do weight training.
- Spend time in nature.
- Journal, write, or make art.
- Engage in music therapy.
- Meditate.
- Eat good, nutritious foods.
- Make time for social outings.

One of my first "cancer buddies" in real life was Rodney, who lived about 30 minutes from my town in Maine. Rodney coped with his cancer by getting outside and hiking when his health allowed. I went for several short hikes and walks with Rodney during the pandemic.

One of the best parts of those hikes was the fact that we rarely talked about cancer. We talked about sports, the New England Patriots and the Boston Celtics mostly. We talked about our dogs and families and the places and people that shaped our lives.

There is tremendous value in simply spending time, especially active time (if possible), with people who are going through the same shitstorm.

Rodney and I were both in the stage IV weeds, going through surgeries and treatment, but we didn't need to talk about it all the time. We needed to NOT talk about it.

Maybe you don't feel like talking about cancer. But you might feel like going to a ballgame, going fishing, or going out for beers with other guys who can identify with what you're facing.

Men crave socialization with other men, but they are nervous about someone forcing them to open up.

You don't need to open up unless you want to. But you do need to get out of your man cave. Sitting there by yourself is not a strategy for health.

I recently prompted my friends online to explain to me and others why taking care of their mental health matters, to share how they do it. These are just a few of the responses.

Seeking help for mental health is a strength, not a weakness. I take care of my mental health by looking for good moments in each day, and if I don't see them in front of me, I create them for others.

– Tom Wallace,
A cancer survivor from Massachusetts

I take care of my mental health by seeing my psychiatrist every two weeks. There's no shame in seeing a doctor for a lung infection, so why would there be shame for taking care of your mind's health?

– David De Wilde,
A survivor from Belgium

I take care of my mental health by keeping physically active—hiking, rucking, weight training, skiing, cycling. Keep moving, whatever your abilities.

– Brian Smith,
A survivor from upstate New York

TAKE PART IN THE PATIENT-TO-PATIENT MOVEMENT

About a year into my cancer journey, I was interested in learning about clinical trials. I consulted with a few doctors at a major cancer center in the Northeast. They talked about the trials available at their center. They were smart and kind, and they let me know they did not have any clinical trials currently that matched my criteria, but there could be some coming in the future.

I thought this meant there were no clinical trials for me ANYWHERE. What I didn't realize is that they were only telling me about the options at their institution.

It was not part of their practice to go the extra mile, to explore with me the trials that I might be eligible for at other cancer centers, like Johns Hopkins, MD Anderson, Duke University, or City of Hope.

And I'm not blaming them at all. They weren't being malicious. At large cancer centers, many doctors don't even have the bandwidth to know the trials available at their own hospital, let alone the thousands of trials available elsewhere.

It's also a matter of business. Cancer centers are designed to keep you as a patient, so you don't need to go elsewhere. These centers can feel like silos, cut off from one another in many ways.

I'm not saying doctors withhold information that could help their patients; they simply don't have the time and resources required to search clinical trials all day long, for each individual patient.

When I told my friends in Colontown that I had struck out looking for trials at the one major cancer center, they bombarded me with high quality information about trials at other centers that matched my disease criteria.

As I said earlier, I had thought I would learn the most about my disease and my treatment options from my medical providers. As it turned out, I have learned the most from other patients who have walked the same road.

Most types of cancer have national or international organizations that advocate for awareness, public policy changes, and treatment advances. Those organizations usually have online communities, which is where the patient-to-patient movement lives. Your job is to find the best, most trusted, most reliable communities, and then to dive in.

Julie Saliba Clauer, whom I mentioned in Chapter 6, was diagnosed with stage IV colorectal cancer in March of 2018, the same month and year in which I was diagnosed. She was 43 years old then, and her daughter was only seven months old. Julie has since navigated her journey with the help of Colontown and now serves on its leadership team, focusing on patient education.

Julie interviewed seven oncologists in her quest for the right person who could extend her life and give her more time with her husband and daughter. She moved from Chicago to California to be under the care of one of the world's top medical oncologists, Dr. Heinz-Josef Lenz at the University of Southern California.

By combining traditional techniques with a cutting-edge clinical trial, Julie has far outlived her initial prognosis.

Before cancer, Julie spent her life immersed in the languages of food, travel, and marketing. When she was diagnosed with colorectal cancer that had spread to her liver, she googled, "Where is my liver?" I was in that same boat when I was diagnosed. I remember googling, "Where is my colon, and what does it do?"

"I was medically and scientifically clueless," Julie recalled. "I lined up an incredible care team. But it was Colontown where I learned the language and how to navigate all things cancer. From my fellow patients, I became familiar with clinical trials from watching them and asking questions when I was confused. I got a humanized crash course in scientific research, treatment strategy, personal decision making, and statistics. All of this enabled me to have meaningful conversations about clinical trials with my oncologist, reach out effectively to primary investigators on other trials of interest, and make well informed treatment decisions."

Armed with her new language, Julie now gives back so much to Colontown and the larger colorectal cancer community. She spends much of her time educating other patients about treatment options and clinical trials.

Just because you are not an oncologist doesn't mean you can't learn about cancer and take an active role in your treatment.

If you hire an architect, you can learn plenty about architecture and design, to the point that you can collaborate with the architect. It's your house, right?

If you hire a lawyer for a business dispute, you can learn plenty about the law, to the point that you can collaborate with your lawyer. It's your business, right?

The same principle applies to oncology. Yet we are made to think that we should just take a back seat, do what the doctor tells us, and don't rock the boat. That is an old-school, patriarchal model of cancer care. There are still plenty of people who would tell us that we are just patients. They say we aren't smart enough to understand medicine.

Do not be intimidated. No matter what your education or background, you can absolutely learn enough about your disease to play an active role in your care. If you struggle with the learning, find family members, friends, or advocates who will stand up with you. If your oncologist doesn't want your input, fire them.

It's your life on the line, and you have the absolute right to be involved in the decisions around your care. Period.

PLAY

Outside of spending time with family, friends, and of course Grace the dog, my favorite activity during cancer has been mountain biking.

Right around the time of my first liver surgery, I bought a 2011 Scott Genius, full-suspension, black-frame bike with many dings and scratches...and a glinting gold chain.

There have been lots of times during chemotherapy, immunotherapy, and surgery recoveries when mountain biking is not possible. But when I feel good enough, I ride as much as I can. I'm not talking about anything really difficult. I don't do a lot of uphill climbing. I'm not skilled enough to do technical trails with lots of rocks and all that stuff. I'm talking about simple, flowing trails through the woods here in Maine.

I love pushing my body, feeling my heart working, and getting a good sweat going. When I'm able to cruise through the birches, oaks, and pine trees; then power uphill over roots; and coast down a slope with the breeze in my face— that is absolute bliss.

There is no cancer when I'm on my bike. Just my mind, body, and bike focusing on the trail winding out in front of me. If you allow your mind to drift, you can get hurt.

The cancer journey can be so damn heavy. Play is essential.

If all you do is immerse yourself in the planning, the research, the cancer community, the treatment options, etc., you run the risk of missing out on joy. I strongly encourage all cancer patients to find at least one activity that connects them to the concept of play.

There are plenty of options for playfulness. I've been lucky that I've been physically able to bike, hike, and do other activities that fall into the category of play. I'm also aware that many of my friends have serious physical limitations. For them, play is done through video games, board games, arts and crafts, community theater, and so much more. One of the members of the Howling Place group is now doing stand-up comedy.

I asked members of the Howling Place to describe the role of play in their cancer journeys. I would love to share the 20+ answers I received, but I had to pick three.

I hooked up a Nintendo Classic (new HDMI version with preloaded games) illegally to the TV in the infusion center. I played Dr. Mario, Galaga, and Super Mario Brothers during my last three months of chemo. My scores got better when chemo was going in. Really helped to inject laughter into the situation and nurses would check in on the scores. Still play to this day, and I want to think it helps my brain make connections.

– Matthew Parker, Virginia,
Metastatic male breast cancer

Play can mean different things to different folks. Of course I like to meet up with the guys to watch a ball game, or hang out with the love of my life, but to me, play can be so much more, especially when you are in active treatment. To me, play is taking the time to work on my own mental health. I accomplish this in many ways. If the weather is nice, I take a ride on my bike, go out to photograph nature, or fly my drone. If it's not so nice, I work on producing videos, meditate, or work on one of the many paintings I have "in progress." Learning to be still and tune out all of the stresses that come along with this disease is most important. Creating something beautiful out of an ugly situation is my motivation in life now.

– Jesse Dillon, Colorado,
Stage IVB squamous cell carcinoma of the tonsil

Throughout my cancer journey I found a new meaning for play and its importance and healing nature. I would get goofy with my dog, be crazy-fun "Uncle Jay," and do literally anything for my little nieces! I went as far as taking part in my fire department's "calendar" to fundraise for a local charity (PICC line and all). Let's not forget my flashy, funny socks I used to wear to each chemo session or scan just to get a smile and laugh from the staff!

In October of 2021 I learned a totally new meaning of "play" when my wife and I adopted a beautiful little 12-month-old girl, two weeks after finishing chemo. Living in the moment, laughter, not caring what any-one thinks, and doing what makes you happy are all lessons I relearned from a now 2 year old. Play and getting lost in the moment, deep in laughter, brings so much joy and powerful healing energy.

– Jay Abramovitch, Ontario, Canada,

Stage III colorectal cancer

CHAPTER 12

WALKING EACH OTHER HOME

AS HIDEOUS AS it was, the kitchen sink chemotherapy of 2021 totally paid off. My blood work improved soon after starting treatment, and my CT scans showed dramatic improvement. My oncologists called it a home run.

That was huge, because there was a question as to whether the chemo would work for those persistent peritoneal metastases. After eight cycles, all of my tumors had shrunk down to the point where I was eligible for surgery.

I interviewed three potential surgeons and ultimately decided to go with Dr. James Cusack, director of the Peritoneal Surface Malignancy Program at Massachusetts General Hospital in Boston. When someone runs a laboratory with their name on it, usually that's a pretty good choice.

Dr. Cusack is intense in that scholarly way; he's quick witted, kind, meticulous, and aggressive in his approach to surgery. He's the kind of man who probably would have been flying jets if he hadn't decided to treat cancer.

He also loves that I'm an educated, empowered patient

who shows up to meetings with notes, questions, ideas, and always ready to attack the problem. During our first meeting I started talking to him about some clinical trials that explore the connection between colorectal cancer and the gut microbiome.

He put his hand to his chin and said, "What is it again that you do?"

"Well, I was trained as a journalist and worked as a news reporter for many years. Now I spend most of my time running a cancer support organization…and trying to stay alive."

"A journalist," he said, smiling. "You're the people who corner me at parties with your questions. Well, what have you got for me today?"

That was the start to a beautiful doctor–patient relationship. We take the time to understand one another and clarify any confusion. And we always leave our meetings agreeing on a plan. I've had the same experience with his colleague, Dr. Jeff Clark, a medical oncologist who is the director of clinical trials support at Mass General.

I have been incredibly fortunate that Dr. Cusack and Dr. Clark bring their combined experience, knowledge, and talents to my care, to supplement the excellent care I receive from my local oncologist, Dr. Devon Evans at New England Cancer Specialists.

CANCER AS A CHRONIC ILLNESS

In September of 2021, I underwent a cytoreductive surgery (CRS), also known as debulking. Dr. Cusack and his team members removed all the visible cancer from my abdomen plus small portions of my stomach, liver, and spleen. I was in surgery for about seven hours.

Recovery from that one was rough but manageable. When I recurred with a few small tumors in early 2022, I had a second CRS. That recovery was easy; I was walking two miles a day within one week of surgery.

My cancer has behaved strangely, in a good way. Yes, it keeps recurring, so that hasn't been great, but the new tumors have been popping up in the same area of my abdomen.

We think my prior immunotherapy, plus the chemotherapy, have prevented the disease from spreading to other organs or regions of my body. For most people this far into the journey with metastatic disease, surgery is no longer an option.

Our plan is to use surgery as long as we can, with occasional systemic therapy to bridge the gaps. Some patients call this playing "whack-a-mole." Dr. Cusack calls it "berry picking." After many years of battling, it's a fantastic place to be, and I'm grateful.

Unless you know me, you would never guess I'm living

with stage IV cancer. But I feel all of it. My feet are about 30 percent numb from one of my chemotherapy drugs. I have persistent pain in my abdomen and digestive problems caused by adhesions from the surgeries. My skeleton feels like it has aged 50 years in the past five. I have a low-level tremor from PTSD.

I'm in that scary category that some call "terminal." I much prefer the term I learned from Dr. Tom Marsilje: "currently incurable."

There may not be a cure for me right now, but I have been successful at extending my life by using a variety of tools and managing my cancer as a chronic illness. And for those of us who can keep extending the timeline, it's entirely possible that the next big breakthrough is just around the corner. I always remind myself that immunotherapy was not even used in humans until 2006, and that breakthrough has extended and saved thousands of lives just in the past few decades.

Dr. Cusack tells me to "keep an open mind." I have no problem following that order.

―――――――――――――

COPING WITH LOSS IN CANCER SUPPORT GROUPS

Early in 2022, I received a phone call from a relatively new member of the Howling Place group.

"I need some advice with my therapist," he said. "I've been having a great experience in the group, but she doesn't think the Howling Place is good for me. She thinks cancer support groups are overwhelming and depressing. She asked me how I'm going to handle it when I get close to these new friends and then they die."

I tried to collect my thoughts. First off, our cancer group is anything but depressing. In fact, we have a blast most of the time. Secondly, we only have two options as patients and survivors: We can participate in groups where we give and receive support with people facing the same struggles, or we can avoid those groups.

I asked the member two questions.

"Does spending time in the Howling Place help ease the burden of cancer for you?"

"Yes," he said.

"Are you ready to confront the reality of mortality, for yourself, and for the people you love?" I asked him.

"Yes," he said.

"Then I think you need to have an honest conversation with your therapist," I said. "You can keep it simple. Tell her that the happiness you get from your relationships with these friends, and the honor of walking them home, outweighs the pain of losing them."

In this member's case, the positives outweighed the drawbacks, so he stayed in the group and has become one of our core contributors.

For some other men who join the Howling Place, it's not the right fit. Some patients don't want to fill their online lives with other people impacted by cancer. Many others are simply not ready to get close to dying people. That is absolutely normal, and individual comfort rules the day. If you come into the group for a while, get something out of it, and move on, we celebrate you.

The goal of Man Up to Cancer has always been to make sure men avoid isolation during the cancer journey. The Howling Place is one tool for doing that, but there are plenty of other ways to connect and avoid isolation.

As our group grew, it was clear that this emotional challenge—coping with the losses of our cancer friends—would need to be discussed and processed as much as possible in the group itself, and on my podcast.

Dennis Wilbur, one of the original members of the group, died in March of 2021. There was an outpouring of love for Dennis in the Howling Place, and also a collective grief.

As much as I could, I composed my thoughts around Dennis' death, and I wrote a journal entry that would become a podcast episode titled "Walking Each Other Home: Friendship and Loss in Cancer Support Groups." We borrow the phrase "walking each other home" from Ram Dass, a teacher and author whose books include 1971's *Be Here Now*.

This is the original journal entry, ending with a poem I wrote about cancer and grief.

> This past week, we lost one of our original members, Dennis Wilbur. Dennis was a fixture in the Howling Place. Always smiling, always supportive, while going through hell. That sideways grin; that dry humor....
>
> As a community, we experience loss in a way that very few communities ever have to face.
>
> Being part of a cancer support community sometimes feels like being in the infantry. You know that you're going to lose a lot of your brothers along the way. This can absolutely be overwhelming sometimes.
>
> So how do we cope?
>
> As a disclaimer, I'm not an expert on grief and loss. But as a patient advocate over the past few years, being active in a number of cancer support communities, I've been forced to come face to face with loss, and with my own mortality, and I hope that I've been learning and evolving through that.
>
> First things first: There is no right or wrong way to cope. Loss hits us all differently. Man Up to Cancer is a zero-judgment zone for this area. Be easy on yourself; take care of yourself.

We are here for you on YOUR terms. As part of our community, you decide what feels supportive and helpful to you…and the times when you need space.

If this is too much for you—if it's overwhelming, de-stabilizing for your mental health—step away from it. That's OK. That is absolutely nothing to feel bad about. Go live your life away from #cancerland, and lean on the community when you need to.

I was absolutely in that place earlier in my own journey. Seeing people with my same disease, literally watching them get sicker and sicker, and then pass away—that can be rattling to the core. I definitely wasn't ready to confront that. I turned away, and that's what I needed to do at the time. Things are different for me now.

Others in the group are in a place where they feel ready to take on the emotional weight, the heavy toll, that comes with the death of a brother, because that is how we feel about each other in the wolfpack. For me and a lot of the members, it really is a family.

So for those who feel prepared, the experience of loss that we go through in the Howling Place can be an opportunity for growth.

It can empower us to realize we have the strength to walk our friends all the way home…and to realize that we have others willing to do the same for us.

Facing the death of a friend with an open heart is also a huge step toward coming to terms with our own mortality and what that means to us. It forces us to grapple with our darkest fear, sadness, anger, uncertainty.

That can be really uncomfortable, sometimes down-right terrifying, but by confronting death face to face we start to take away the power it might have over us. This very personal appraisal of death, ulti-mately, is a healthy step in a man's life.

Some might ask: Why put yourself through such pain? Why be part of a community where you build these loving friendships, knowing that you will be mourning so many losses?

To quote Alfred Lord Tennyson, "'Tis better to have loved and lost, than never to have loved at all."

We are blessed by the friendships we make in our support group. These bonds make us better peo-ple, we avoid the awful consequences of isolation, and our burden is made lighter by sharing it with our community.

And what is the alternative? To avoid friendships out of fear of loss? To bury our heads in the sand and try to avoid the reality that death is where we are all headed? As a person living with cancer, would I want a potential friend to avoid me because of worry about me dying?

What I'm saying is: If we spend our time trying to avoid unpleasant feelings, we also miss out on the relationships that make life worth living.

I'm still in the process of clarifying my own belief system about death, and a lot of that learning is happening thanks to the interactions in the Howling Place group.

For me, coping means I give myself space to feel and process that grief, and then I honor those guys by living with as much love and joy and purpose as I can, for as long as I can.

When it's my time to go, that is absolutely what I would want for the people I leave behind, including every member of the wolfpack.

I imagine all of the people I've lost cheering me on and telling me to LIVE my life to the fullest. That is how I honor them best.

Jared McMillan introduced me to the concept of picking up their banners and carrying them forward. They are relying on us to do that for them.

This mindset doesn't dull the hardship of loss, but that's how I keep moving forward.

I want the men of the Howling Place to know that the death of our brothers will not diminish our capacity to love and to celebrate life.

Instead, it will enhance that capacity.

Another way to honor Dennis is to help ease the burden for another member of the group. Respond to a post, give encouragement, even if it's just a few words, get involved in some of the conversations. What better way to honor the departed than to spend some time every day helping someone else.

The Man Up to Cancer community means the world to me. I get goosebumps every time I think about going to battle with you guys.

Remember that all of us—the guys who have passed and those of us who pick up their banners—are better off for the time we spent supporting one another.

When I think of that phrase "walking each other home," it is the privilege of a lifetime to help ease the burden of the walk…and to have others walking me home, too.

The genuine love and care that we see every day in the Howling Place is astounding and it really, really matters.

Because we can all get caught up in the day-to-day,

trivial stuff in life—the small upsets, the hard feelings, the drudgery and responsibility.

But at the end of the day, as human beings, we all want to know that we are cared for, that we are valued, and that we are loved, even in our sickness... and all the way to our death.

It takes courage to see each other all the way down the path.

There is no lack of courage in the Howling Place, and I'm incredibly proud of that.

I love you guys. KFG.

CANCER AND GRIEF
BY TREVOR MAXWELL

Grief shows up at your door and you want to turn it away

Because you know how much it's going to hurt.

Yet you also know it won't leave you alone until you spend time with it.

Grief visits on its own, non-negotiable terms.

These recent days have been grieving kind of days.

It has come into the house of my heart and made itself quite comfortable.

My limbs are heavy, my brain caught in cycles of the same sad thoughts.

Grief for the battered landscape of my own mind and body.

For what my wife and daughters have endured over the past four years.

For the friends I have lost and will continue to lose.

Grief for the irretrievable time I have spent fighting, under threat of death, when cancer has had me cornered and I'm stripped down to the singular instinct of survival.

Grief for a society full of thoughts and prayers and little action, a complacency that would profit forever from our poisoning, burning, and cutting.

Grief for the children left behind, and the children facing a grown person's fight.

Grief at knowing that while I have laid down my sword for the past few months, I will almost certainly be called again to that brutal and bloody field.

And still, I must rally and stand against despair.

I must know that grief is a visitor, not a permanent resident here.

Grief will move along. In the very writing of this, I sense its restlessness.

And in the morning, maybe tomorrow even, a kinder visitor will come.

Maybe hope, or gratitude.

Perhaps even joy.

CHAPTER 13

FAMILY

POEM TO SARAH from your husband

Mother's Day, May 11, 2008

Thank you for Sage
    Our dreamer
    Our moon reacher
        Little arms stretching skyward
Brown eyes
The one who peeked at us and smiled
The one who still peeks and smiles
        Or reaches a soft hand without looking
        To feel our warmth, still close
            Our kitchen floor jumper
            Our rhythmic dancer
            Our book sleeper
Every day of her life
You have brought her joy and sustenance and knowledge
            Our water tester
She will come to the edge of the surf and step beyond
When she is ready

Thank you for Elsie

    Our fearless one

    Our smile giver

        Little arms and legs churning forward

    Blue eyes

    The one who climbed us sleeping like mountains

    The one who still climbs and throws hands around our necks

        And roars her delight

        With an all-cheeks grin

            Our loud girl waiting for words

            Our leap taker

            Our reluctant sleeper

    Every day of her life

    You have brought her joy and sustenance and knowledge

        Our quick diver

    She will pause to speak our names

    When she is ready

Thank you for you

    My best companion

    My wife reflected in two beautiful daughters

Moon reacher and smile giver

    The one who calms and supports and sacrifices

    The one who runs and goes to the gym and finds strength through yoga

And takes the dazzling photographs

That capture us all in time

My caregiver

My squash sponsor

My lover for now and forever

Every day of my life

You have brought me joy and sustenance and knowledge

My Sarah

You will fully know the strength of your mother-spirit

When you are ready

I wrote that poem for Sarah nearly 15 years ago. I was 31, she was 30. Sage was just about to turn 3 years old, and Elsie was almost 1.

Through all the intervening years, including nearly five of them living with cancer, they are still those same people. I want to tell you about each of them.

For a man who was diagnosed with stage IV cancer at age 41, when it comes to my family, I still feel like I'm the luckiest guy in the world.

SAGE

Sage is 17 now, a high school senior, and she is coming into her own as a smart, kind, funny, and talented young woman. She is still a dreamer. After being tentative and shy for most of her childhood, just over the past few years she has begun to share her gifts with others. In our small town, she is known best for her beautiful singing voice.

For years, I would listen to her sing in the house and say, "When are you going to show the world your talent?"

She just wasn't ready yet. Then, the amazing Ms. Lee, the high school choral director, finally convinced Sage to take a solo part. Probably 30 people came up to me afterward: "Oh my goodness, we didn't know Sage could sing like that!" Then the word was out. Sports teams started asking her to sing the national anthem at games, and she crushed every single performance.

Sage was even asked to sing the anthem at the start of the Beach To Beacon road race, which draws runners from around the world to our town. In front of more than 7,000 participants, including the race founder—Maine native and winner of the first women's Olympic marathon in 1984, Joan Benoit Samuelson—Sage sang with confidence and heart and didn't miss a note.

In the fall of 2023, Sage plans on attending college, most likely the University of Maine. She is considering speech language pathology as a career path. No matter what she chooses, the field will be lucky to have her.

ELSIE

Elsie is 15, a high school sophomore who gets a ride to school most days from her older sister. Notice I didn't say big sister. That's because Elsie is about four inches taller and has been bigger than Sage since the early days. Elsie is still fearless. We could airdrop her to some country halfway around the world and she would learn a new language, find a host family, get a job, and save enough money to come back home.

When Elsie is around the house, you can't miss her. She stomps like me, and she speaks her mind with passion and an undeniable engagement in life.

The biggest problem Elsie faces is that she wants to do it all. Just this year, she is participating in Model United Nations, World Affairs Council, Women's Union Council, botany club, robotics, volleyball, indoor track, softball, and probably other clubs she hasn't told me about because she knows I'll tell her it's too much.

Elsie has played on a softball travel team since she was 8 years old. The sport has taken us all over New England as well as to South Carolina, Georgia, and Florida. It has taught her invaluable life lessons such as teamwork, leadership, work ethic, humility, how to celebrate success, and how to cope with failure.

Elsie is already dreaming about the possibility of going somewhere fun, new, and challenging for college, maybe on the West Coast. Of course, when the time approaches things could change. But her adventurous spirit has been clear since the beginning, and I expect that will last forever.

SARAH

Sarah stole my heart when we were teenagers, and I haven't yet asked for it back.

We were just kids then, sneaking around to spend time together, writing each other funny notes in physics class. I would never have believed you if you had told me we would get married, have two kids, and build our lives together.

Thankfully, that's how it happened.

Sarah has blue-green-yellow eyes that change with the weather and with the colors she's wearing. She is practical, grounded, and organized, while also loving travel and adventure. If I need to figure out a gift for someone, I ask Sarah because she always comes up with the best ideas, thinking of small ways to make everyone feel special. I figured out early on that she has both a superhuman sense of hearing and smell, along with long-distance eyesight. You may not ever know it, but she sees everything.

Sarah has made a career as a public school teacher, administrator, and curriculum expert. She is an exceptionally hard worker who cares deeply for the students at her school. She doesn't like the spotlight and recognition, but I'm not the only person who recognizes that Sarah is an all-star at her job.

Facing a life-threatening disease in the prime of our lives was certainly not the plan. It's not what I envisioned for her.

Honestly, I have the easy part. I go through the treatments and the surgeries. I know it has been harder on Sarah, and I would sacrifice anything to take away one ounce of that struggle. I know my cancer wasn't my fault, but occasionally I still have feelings of guilt. Other families around us are planning out their futures while every plan we make is shrouded by uncertainty.

I have had to adjust to the unfamiliar role of "patient," and Sarah has had to adjust to the equally unfamiliar role she was thrust into—"caregiver."

It hasn't been a Hallmark movie. During the first year, when I fell into my mental health pit, Sarah would get angry and resentful because I was "checked out." I would get angry and resentful because she couldn't understand my experience, and I hated being dependent. I felt like damaged goods.

There have been fights, frustrations, and periods of emotional distance. My loss of confidence, physically and emotionally, made me withdraw. Sarah has withdrawn out of self protection. How could she keep her heart open and at the same time brace herself for the most likely outcome—losing me?

As it turns out, love is not always roses and date nights.

Sarah has shown me love with her presence in the hospital

waiting rooms; by standing by my bed when I wake up from anesthesia; by texting or calling all our friends and family members with updates; by walking the hallways with me when I was hooked up to countless tubes and monitors, making sure my urine container didn't spill or I didn't accidentally run over the tubes.

After my first surgery, when they took out 20 inches of my colon and reconnected the healthy sections, I was sick and in tremendous pain for three or four days before my digestive system learned how to function again. When that happened, we hugged and cried in the hospital bathroom.

No, it's not sexy. But for us, two people who've relied on each other for most of our lives, that's what love looks like sometimes. It's messy and raw and beautiful.

Through it all, we have made the daily choice to love one another and to raise our children— to celebrate them together. There is nothing better than meeting up with Sarah to watch a chorus concert or a softball game, where these little humans we created go out and do their thing.

Laughter has sometimes been hard to come by. I'd say that both of us, in part because of our backgrounds and stuff we went through as kids, tend toward serious moods. We have been conscious about inserting "play" back into our lives, but I'm the first to admit that the heaviness of cancer affects me. That makes it even sweeter when Sarah and I share a laughing fit.

One day in 2020, when I was on immunotherapy, I stayed in bed most of the day because I didn't feel quite right.

My face and hands felt super tingly, and my vision seemed a little strange.

When Sarah got home from work, she came in to check on me.

"Uh, are you OK?" she asked.

"I think so. I just feel funny," I answered.

"Have you looked at your face? I think you need to look at your face," she said.

So I got up and walked into the bathroom. My face was so swollen, I hardly recognized myself. Apparently the immunotherapy had gone rogue, causing inflammation in my eyelids, cheeks, and lower jaw. I turned to Sarah, who was standing beside me looking concerned.

"I look like Quasimodo!" I said, and we both started cracking up. "Turn away, I'm hideous!" I said, acting out the part of the outcast hunchback.

A strong dose of prednisone calmed the inflammation. We laughed about that scene for weeks.

I give myself 10 percent credit for keeping us intact as a family. Sarah gets the rest.

As I said earlier in this book, there was a time early on in my cancer journey when I practically begged Sarah to let me go. Sarah's family owns a remote camp in the wilderness of northern Maine, and I wanted to go there by myself, where my cancer would be mine alone, and I wouldn't be a burden on my family.

Sarah refused. Instead of letting me go, she carried me. She carried all of us during that time, because the girls were much younger. She took care of the household, and the girls, all while working a stressful job to make sure we had income and health insurance. She even finished her master's degree in educational leadership.

As the girls grew, we cobbled together our old traditions and routines, added in some new ones, and created our new normal.

Because of these three people, I was able to make a remarkable comeback, reestablish my roles as husband and father, and help others with the Man Up to Cancer mission.

Things may look different now than they did before cancer, but in some ways, our lives are richer than they were. All I really wanted was a chance for redemption, to show my wife and girls that life will knock you down, but you can get up and do something that matters. They gave me the gift of seeing it through.

The bottom line is this: I wouldn't be alive without the love of Sarah, Sage, and Elsie.

REDEFINING HOPE

My experience with cancer redefined how I view courage.

It also redefined how I view hope.

When you become an adult you have adult hopes. Many of us hope to find a job we enjoy that can pay the bills; love; healthy children; and maybe even an opportunity to make a difference in the world. And if you get sick—if you get cancer—you hope to be cured.

As someone who has lived more than four years with metastatic cancer, gone through five major abdominal surgeries, and had dozens of rounds of chemotherapy and immunotherapy, I have been forced to confront the reality that my hope for a cure might not be in the stars for me.

In the wake of my most recent surgery, in June of 2022, my blood tests showed that I still had some active disease. A CT scan confirmed one new, very small tumor near my pancreas and some enlarging lymph nodes that may also harbor cancer. At this point, it's not surprising. With these surgeries, we are not trying to cure my cancer. Sure, it would be incredible if that happened. Instead, the goal is to reset the clock on my cancer—to extend my life.

With this latest information, I'm circling and weighing my options with my local oncologist, my surgeon and oncologist at Mass General, and my incredibly smart network of patients and other medical providers who are now friends.

We are managing my cancer as a chronic illness, and the name of the game is life extension, while maintaining the best quality of life possible.

So, what does this all have to do with hope?

Back in 2018 and 2019, my concept of hope was simple. I hoped to "beat cancer." That was the popular-culture language available to me at the time. "Beat cancer!" "Kick its ass!" "Cancer picked on the wrong dude!" "You got this!" Cancer was like one of those carnival games on the midway and no matter how many people failed before me, I was going to win.

And it's OK to be in that place. There's nothing wrong with that version of hope, or the people telling me to hope for it. My doctors, nurses, and all the people cheering me on all have the best intentions. When people say, "You're gonna beat this," that is their way of supporting me.

So there I was at the beginning of this journey, facing stage IV colon cancer, where less than 15 percent of patients survive five years beyond the diagnosis, and cure was the only acceptable outcome. I stepped into the ring and started punching.

I had part of my colon removed, then went for a liver surgery we hoped would cure me. My cancer recurred, and I was crushed.

I went for a second liver surgery we hoped would cure me. I recurred; I was crushed.

I blamed myself. I thought, "There's something I'm not doing right. If I could only think or pray the right way, I could be cured, I could win this game."

Of course that seems ridiculous to me now.

Immunotherapy was supposed to be my ace in the hole. I progressed, and I was crushed.

That was when the concept of hope really started to evolve for me.

The concept of hope for a cure was not gone; it was just moving toward the horizon, further and further out of reach.... I was slowly realizing that, in all likelihood, cancer will take my life at some point, unless a new treatment emerges or I hit the jackpot with a clinical trial. The idea that I would live to see my grandchildren; well, that started to take up less of my thinking.

This was not a naive transition for me. In the past few years, I have lost more than 100 cancer friends. These were strong, brave, loving people who did everything right, and still they died.

Some of you may be thinking, "Well, this is depressing. It must be awful to go through cancer and to lose hope that you'll be cured."

Some of you may even be thinking that I'm not going to reach a cure if I don't hold a singular belief that it's going to happen for me.

All I can say is this: You haven't walked in my shoes.

I still have hope for a long life. It just doesn't take up a lot of my time—time that is far better spent living in the moment rather than being so attached to one outcome.

When I spend time on hope nowadays, I hope for things that are grounded in the here and now. I hope for tomorrow to be the best possible day for me and my family.

I hope the weather agrees tomorrow so I can take Grace the dog for our usual walk around Great Pond, where a light mist might be moving through the reeds on the water. I hope we have a blast on the camping trip we're taking this week.

I hope that when my time does come that I will be remembered as kind.

I hope Sarah and I will get to sit on the porch and watch as the colors turn from green to gold, then orange, yellow, and brown this fall, and again next fall if Mother Nature sees it fitting.

I hope the Red Sox have a better season next year.

I'm not suggesting that it's a mistake to hope you find a cure. That would be cruel and hypocritical. I still want that, too.

I just don't think it's helpful or wise to fixate on a singular hope, especially when we do not have as much control over the situation as some of us cancer patients would like to believe.

If you look at cancer as an opponent to beat, and plan to get back to living when you're cured, what happens if that cure never comes?

What if you go years clinging to that one hope that never gets answered, so much so that outside the treatments and the surgeries you've numbed yourself out of the life that's right in front of you. What if you're sleepwalking?

If you spend long enough in Cancerland, you know people like this. They're still living, but they're so consumed with beating cancer that they aren't really engaged in the present—and many are in denial. They never really confront what it means to live and to die—to be human—until it's too late.

So go ahead and remain hopeful for your cure, and I will as well. Just please don't lose sight of the day-to-day living.

For those of us who will ultimately die from cancer, there is still deep meaning in our existence. There is still beauty. There is still wonder and awe, even if our lives are not to be as long as we, or our loved ones, had imagined.

CHAPTER 14

THE GATHERING
OF WOLVES

FROM THE BEGINNING, the Howling Place wasn't just another Facebook group. It wasn't just another cancer support group.

It was, and always will be, a brotherhood.

For the men who really vibe with the people and the environment, it's a place we go to share the burden of cancer and to celebrate the big and small joys of living. It's one place that we have, just for us, where we don't feel like misfits, sick people, or outcasts. We crack up at each other's memes; we hold each other up when the scans are not good or when relationships get rocky; and we're there for each other when we need to rage.

Social media gave us the platform and tools to find one another, to build these relationships through posts, comments, private messages, and Zoom meetings.

For those who are able to meet up in person, that's where the brotherhood goes to the next level. Small meet-ups happen all the time.

186

Members of the Howling Place have gotten together in places like New York City, Minneapolis, Washington, DC, as well as North Carolina, Florida, Texas, and elsewhere. I remember one photo in particular in which Michael "Mike" Riehle and Mat Monte-De Vito met up in a hallway at Memorial Sloan Kettering Cancer Center in NYC, both wearing their hospital gowns and grinning from ear to ear.

Early on, Joe Bullock and I talked a lot about holding an event where we could bring the whole group together, but the coronavirus pandemic and the setbacks of my own cancer battle made that impossible.

In the spring of 2022, I made the decision that it was time to have an in-person event.

However, I was too overwhelmed to plan it myself. I was still facing active cancer, raising teenage daughters, doing the podcast, working as a consultant for two health tech companies, and focusing on raising the profile of Man Up to Cancer (MUTC) so I could fundraise for the gathering as well as our Chemo Backpack program. (Joe Bullock and I had started sending out backpacks each month filled with comfort items and practical gifts for men in the MUTC community going through chemotherapy.)

One night, I was venting to Sarah that I couldn't do all of this. Once again, she saw the simple truth I couldn't see.

"Uh, you don't need to plan the event yourself," she said. "You have hundreds of guys in your group. I'm sure there

187

are some who want to be involved more. You can do the fundraising, and choose the right guys for the job."

Cue the lightbulb. I already knew who I would ask. The only question I had was, would they accept the challenge?

The next day, I sent a private message to Don Helgeson (colorectal, prostate, melanoma, from Nanaimo, BC, Canada); Michael Riehle (colorectal, South Wales, NY); and Danny Riggs (male breast cancer, Houston, TX). I asked if they could have a Zoom meeting with me that night. I fooled them into thinking there was a problem in the Howling Place that we needed to discuss.

When we were all on the meeting, I said, "You know how we've all been wanting to do a big gathering for the group? Well, you guys are planning it!"

They were both shocked and relieved. They thought I was pissed off about something and they were being called into the principal's office.

Of course, I didn't force anyone to plan the gathering. I told them they could only do the planning if it fit into their lives, if their spouses approved, and if it would bring them a sense of fulfillment. I would raise all the money to fund the gathering; they could even use some of the money to hire a planner to help them. Danny Riggs, unbeknownst to me, had experience planning large events. He said they wouldn't need to hire a pro.

"Hold my beer" were his exact words.

Fortunately for the Howling Place, Don, Mike, and Danny were the absolute perfect team for the mission (and Sara Riehle; I'm not forgetting you!). Over the next six months they planned and executed the best, and perhaps the largest, retreat ever held for men impacted by all types of cancer. I could go on here, but let's just say this: They worked their asses off, and I'm forever grateful.

More than 50 members of the group attended the inaugural Gathering of Wolves, also known as GOW, held in September of 2022 at Camp Duffield in Delevan, NY, just south of Buffalo. Several other members intended to go but could not because of stupid cancer.

Having been in the group for two and a half years, I knew the quality of these guys, and I was expecting magic. But even I was not prepared for the level of openness, selflessness, and camaraderie on display at Camp Duffield.

I'm not going to attempt to describe the GOW from start to finish because you don't need to hear it all and I can't even capture it.

It was a blur of hugs, laughter, tears, endless conversations, cornhole, campfires, music, food, and drink.

So I'm going to share with you some fragments of memory, and then I'll share some words from a few members who were also there, Jason Manuge and David De Wilde.

STEVEN BARKER: THIS IS
YOUR WEEKEND, TOO

The day before the gathering, we held a pre-party at Mike and Sara Riehle's house, which is about a 30-minute drive from Camp Duffield. Mike and Sara were the most generous hosts one could ever imagine. Throughout the afternoon and evening, members of the Howling Place arrived from all across the U.S. and Canada. I knew almost all of them from the group, and it was such a joy to meet them in person.

It was also surreal. I could feel my anxiety creeping in, and I knew where it was coming from. As the founder of Man Up to Cancer, I felt responsible for their weekend. They had left their families and responsibilities to come to New York because of a mission that I had started. What if the event fell flat? What if they didn't enjoy themselves?

I could feel myself sinking under the burden. Thankfully, my buddy from Memphis, Steven Barker, pulled me aside. We spent about 15 minutes talking, one-on-one, on the front lawn. I told him about the burden of responsibility that I was feeling.

"Man, that's totally understandable. I know you want everyone to have a great time," Steven said. "But this is your weekend, too. Just like you are here for us, we are here for you. So take that pressure off yourself."

That was exactly what I needed to hear. Throughout the weekend, I remained attentive to the needs of others but not at the expense of myself. I made sure my cup was filled.

CANNONBALLS #TOLIFE

Whenever I have a chance to swim, to jump in a pool, pond, lake, or ocean, I try to take advantage of that opportunity. It's calming and energizing at the same time.

And if I get a chance to cannonball, you better believe that's happening.

Dr. Tom Marsilje, the legendary patient and cancer researcher whose writings taught me so much about my disease and my mindset, always did cannonballs while shouting his slogan "To Life!"

So when I saw the pristine pond that Mike and Sara had created in their backyard, I seized the moment, stripped down to my boxers, and took the cannonball leap. Danny snapped a photo of me in midair. The next day, at Camp Duffield, I did the same thing at the pond there. That time, I was joined by my friends Alek and Chris.

PINEAPPLE PIZZA WARS: A TRUCE?

One of the longest running debates within the Howling Place revolves around a critical question that all men need to confront: Does pineapple belong on pizza?

I'm in the camp of the purists. Don't get that pineapple anywhere near my pie.

Sadly, about half of the group seems to enjoy this culinary abomination.

People outside of the Howling Place imagine that in our online conversations we're deep in talks about cancer, when really we are exchanging hilarious memes about pineapple pizza! I mean, things have really gotten heated over this.

During the planning of the gathering, I made a foolish promise. I said I would eat pineapple pizza if we could get more than 50 members to attend. Oops. Joe Bullock, who is on the correct side of the pizza war with me, made the same deal.

On Saturday at the gathering, a fresh, hot, pineapple pizza was delivered to Camp Duffield. In front of everyone, Joe and I took our first bites. In a flash, I turned around and tossed my slice into the pond, to the horror of Danny Riggs and the other pineapple-pizza lovers. But then I actually ate a whole slice, and you know what? It didn't kill me.

Are the pizza wars over? Let's just say there's an uneasy truce. But I can't promise not to ignite that feud again.

TEAM CANADA VS. TEAM USA

When it comes to lawn games, cornhole has been the most popular pastime over the last decade or so. Mike Riehle made some custom Man Up to Cancer cornhole boards specifically to unveil at the GOW.

As word spread about the boards, we started to hear some trash talk from our friends up north. The Canadian contingent has been steadily growing in the Howling Place, led in British Columbia by Robby Burridge, Don Helgeson, and Greg Brown; and in eastern Canada by Jay Abramovitch, Gary Puppa, and Jason Manuge.

Don and Greg let the group know that Team Canada was practicing and ready to win at cornhole. For Team USA, Mike Riehle was doing much of the trash talking, along with Gary Bledsoe, who loves to stir the pot (and doesn't even play cornhole).

Mike posted a photo of himself practicing with the caption, "Getting dialed in for the big USA vs. CAN cornhole match coming up in a few weeks. Twenty years from now this is the only thing ESPN will be talking about!"

It was a hotly contested match, and the Americans tried to make a comeback, but in the end the cornhole title went to Team Canada (Don and Greg). They have one year to savor it because I know Team USA will be ready for GOW '23.

JEFF PHILLIPS' 10,000-MILE JOURNEY, ONE STEP AT A TIME

Jeff Phillips is a remarkable human being. He is a stage

IV lung cancer survivor from Rancho Santa Margarita, California.

When he was undergoing treatment, Jeff started walking, and he pretty much never stopped. He would walk a few miles a day at first, and it didn't take long before he was walking 10 or 20 miles at a time.

"I went to see my oncologist," Jeff told me. "We could see the treatment was working. I was feeling better. The cancer was shrinking. He told me, 'Jeff, things are looking good. Just keep doing what you're doing.'"

So he kept walking, and the miles piled up by the thousands. Eventually, Jeff was declared NED (No Evidence of Disease). By then, in the months leading up to the Gathering of Wolves, Jeff was closing in on 10,000 miles of walking. He talked to the event planners, and they decided Jeff would walk that final mile at the gathering, with all of the participants who could walk that last mile with him.

On Saturday morning at GOW, we came together to walk with Jeff. Making the moment even sweeter, one of our leaders, Jay Abramovitch, had the idea to create an actual banner honoring the members of the Howling Place who had passed away.

Surrounded by our wolfpack, Jay handed over the banner to Jeff, who then led us on the final mile of his 10,000-mile trek.

I get goosebumps just writing about it.

———

JASON MANUGE

Jason Manuge, a stage III colorectal cancer patient from Kingston, Ontario, Canada, summed up his thoughts about the GOW in a blog post. I was so moved by what he wrote that I want to share parts of his post with you.

> The profound, transcendent effect this will have on my life will not be adequately communicated through words and pictures, but I'll do my best to give a taste.

> ### Trust and Vulnerability
> So much of the event was centered around people sharing stories and talking about some of the hardest struggles (and funniest moments) we've undergone as a result of our diagnoses. This is, obviously, a very private and personal thing, so I won't betray the trust by sharing details. I will, however, be putting together some of the lessons that I learned from folks over the coming days.

> Conversations ran the gamut from the serious, heavy topics to the lighthearted and fun. But the degree to which we felt comfortable to share with each other was really touching and made the event something special.

> ### Brotherhood
> I truly feel like I understand what it's like to share a revered kinship with a group of people.

195

The closest paradigm I can think of would be a bond between people who've been through the shit together. First responders, soldiers, and the like who are thrust into situations that only those with firsthand experience can understand.

In that way, it's not what's said that makes the bonds strong. It's what doesn't need to be said.

There are three words that ultimately brought us to-gether: You have cancer. And to be around those who've also heard those words is to have an inher-ent understanding.

Through the Gathering, I know that I've strength-ened friendships that will last a lifetime and formed new ones that I will always hold close to my heart.

Perhaps like the bond of soldiers, there is also a somber reminder that some of these friendships may not last long. Cancer, like war, ends lives too soon. It's a very real possibility that some of the men I've come to know and love may not be around for the next Gathering.

That so many people were willing to share the irre-placeable gift of time was really moving.

A Life-changing Experience
Without a doubt, this will be an event that I'll remem-ber for the rest of my life. I can't imagine that anyone

CHAPTER 14: THE GATHERING OF WOLVES

who was able to attend would think differently.

Through great conversations that spanned the gamut of emotions, we reinforced the importance of camaraderie and brotherhood as we all navigate the hellscape of cancer.

These are the types of bonds that will withstand the test of time, help to lift and inspire others, and prove that men—when they allow themselves to be vulnerable—are stronger and better for it.

Hence the Man Up to Cancer motto: Open Heart, Warrior Spirit.

Whatever your current challenge or struggle, just remember to Keep (bleeping) Going."

– Jason Manuge

DAVID DE WILDE

One of the absolute highlights of the Gathering of Wolves was the chance to spend time with David De Wilde, a testicular cancer survivor.

David traveled the farthest to attend the gathering, all the way from Sint-Niklaas, Belgium. Plus, he did it all in a wheelchair. David has neurological disorders, unrelated to his cancer, that severely limit the function of his legs and feet.

He has had numerous surgeries to his legs, hips, and pelvis.

Words cannot capture the indomitable spirit of David De Wilde—the curiosity behind those round-rimmed glasses and the enthusiasm of his hand gestures.

He is a husband, father of two teenagers, researcher and teacher of archaeology and art history, sculptor, chess player, recorder player, and a high-functioning person on the autism spectrum. He had been doing scientific research for many years at Brussels University before his health issues forced him to stop.

Before the GOW, David had never been to the United States. But the bonds he had forged in the Howling Place group compelled him to make the trip.

This is a piece he wrote when the event was over.

NEVER HAD I EVER: A STORY

This seems like a fairy tale, or a bedtime story, or a fantasy…. I find it hard to believe that this trip has actually happened.

Firstly, never had I ever dreamed of having such a supporting wife…. She has been there always, and she is my soulmate, supporting me in all my travels.

Never had I ever, been across the Atlantic

Never had I ever, traveled completely by myself

Never had I ever, traveled as a wheelchair user

Never had I ever, driven in a side-by-side

... yet I was confident in all of this, because I knew I had your support

Never had I ever, eaten waffles with bacon, nor buffalo hot wings, nor hash for breakfast, nor Sarah's amazing chicken dip (was that great or what!), had such amazing grilled chicken, peeps, the food-list goes on....

Never had I ever, had someone waiting for me at the gate of the airport, standing there to welcome and embrace me... a memory I will cherish forever, Danny

Never had I ever, met someone that I admire as much as I do Trevor, for him to take me in his arms as if we had been friends forever, that moment cannot be described

Never had I ever, driven on a strange driveway, feeling I was coming "home"

Never was I ever, as moved at meeting someone so powerful, strong, and loving as you, Joe,

Never had I ever, met a Canadian. Don, you were the very first, and I'm glad it was you

Never had I ever, had the joy of meeting someone with whom I felt an immediate connection. Chris Taylor, that's my shout out to you, my brother

Never had I ever, felt such a profound welcome, such a recognition, such a deep friendship, such an understanding of brotherhood, as when I saw Michael

... by now tears are flowing unstoppable... and

my list is not near long enough; you guys were all amazing

Never had I ever, been the referee of an international competition

Never had I ever, had someone listen to my extremely nerdy archaeology chatter, yes, that's you Jason

Never had I ever, been invited to be a part of such an amazing accomplishment as walking the last of 10,000 miles.

Never had I ever been helped dealing with my disability, where not a single person made me feel as if I needed "special care." Taking me around, bringing my wheelchair, giving me a much-needed push, holding me steady, helping me in the shower or getting dressed... this was just how things were, this was "taking care FOR" a brother without "taking care OF" and everyone made that abundantly clear.

Never had I ever, felt that my disability wasn't a burden to the group but just one single aspect of me

Never had I ever, been on a mens-only retreat, and if you would have told me 6 months ago, I wouldn't have believed you

Never had I ever, seen a quilt, now I have the most precious one in the world! Thank you, Scott, for thinking of me

Never had I ever, had someone give his own backpack to me... a gift out of friendship, it was something no one had ever done for me before

*By now I'm sounding like a poor little sad man,
but that's honestly just the truth of it. I was one
of those men who was down on the floor, and
you reached out and grabbed my hand.*

Never had I ever, been shouted out

*Never had I ever, felt appreciated for who I am, by
"friends".... I didn't realize this, but I had given
up on friendship; I was convinced friendship
just wasn't meant to be for me.... You all proved
me wrong big time. There are simply no words
to describe the warmth, of feeling "valued"*

So...

*Never had I ever, understood the meaning of
friendship*

*Never had I ever, had the honor of reading and
hearing the names of people lost, with tears free-
ly flowing, but also with a fierce determination
to never let someone walk his path alone*

*To say this gathering, this group, was a unique
experience, is selling it short.... It was—in
one word—life changing, more than one could
imagine.*

*Never have I ever, been so fortunate and grateful
to be part of a group, honored to be part of your
lives, humbled to have such wonderful brothers
being part of mine.*

– David De Wilde

To Joe, Don, Michael, Danny, David, and all of my brothers in the Man Up to Cancer community, thank you for loving me and for loving one another.

Along with Sarah, Sage, and Elsie, you have taken me full circle.

My cancer journey started alone, on my living room floor, crying out in despair.

Though my quest to be cancer-free continues, I move forward not alone but with all of your arms around me.

If you read this and I have gone back to the mystery, to the source of all things, take comfort. I'm still with you, and I'm right here in these words, always with an open heart and a warrior spirit.

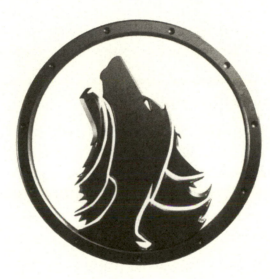

DISCUSSION QUESTIONS

FOR MEN WHO ARE CANCER PATIENTS OR SURVIVORS:

1. How has your own cancer experience been similar to or different from the experiences shared in the book?

2. What do you consider your biggest challenge since being diagnosed with cancer?

3. As a man facing cancer, have you been impacted by isolation? This could be social, physical, or other types of isolation.
   a. If you are no longer isolated, what changed?
   b. If you are still isolated, has this book encouraged you to connect with others?

4. How would you describe your emotional health today?

5. In Chapter 2, the author talks about some of his childhood heroes, and how those characters and athletes shaped some of his early views about manhood. Who were your childhood heroes? Did they influence your views on what it means to be a man in today's world? Are there any behaviors that you have had to question or unlearn?

6. The author experiences two frustrating encounters in Chapter 3, first at a Panera restaurant and then at the bank. Have you faced similar frustrations in your cancer

journey? What emotions did these experiences bring up for you? What did you learn from these emotions?

7. Have you used any of the tips for coping with cancer stress found in Chapter 11?
   a. If so, which ones work best for you?
   b. If not, is there anything holding you back?
   c. Do you have any other healthy coping strategies you would add to the list?

8. Who do you go to when you are experiencing the array of emotions that comes with a cancer diagnosis?

9. How can you make time in your life to prioritize not only your physical but also your mental health?

FOR PEOPLE WHO ARE CAREGIVERS TO A MAN FACING CANCER:

1. What experiences from the book did you relate to from the perspective of being a caregiver?

2. What other experiences from your own life would you add to the discussion about caring for a loved one with cancer?

3. Was there anything from the book that surprised you or stood out?

4. What new understanding or ideas did you take away from the book about how to care for your loved one?

5. What support do you need in order to care for your loved one?

ACKNOWLEDGMENTS

I am the luckiest cancer patient in the world. I have been surrounded by love and support through this entire journey. I am painfully aware that not all patients have this love and support in their lives. To Sarah, Sage, Elsie, my parents, my brother, the Royalls, the Lincolns, my extended family, the Maiers, the Duguays, and our circle of close friends, I could not have done any of this without you.

Joe Bullock, you are the heart of the Howling Place, and I'm forever grateful to be your brother.

Michael Riehle, Don Helgeson, Danny Riggs, and the rest of the MUTC admins and wolfpack leaders (too many to name), you know how I feel about all of you.

Kelin Welborn, you took this concept and gave it a visual identity. Danielle Derbenti, my project manager, you were always the only person for the job. Kim King, you completed our dragonfly squad.

I'm going to make a list here of others who have had an impact on my life and journey. There are additional chapters in my head about all of you, but I hope this thank you will suffice. And to those I have not named, you know you're in my heart.

Patrick Dempsey, J.J. Singleton, Tracy Morgan, Jay Carter, Dave Nitsche, Kevin Gillespie, Carole Motycka and the late Michael Mancini, the late Dr. Tom Marsilje, Sara Riehle, Bob Riehle, Jason Randall, Tom Wallace, David De Wilde, Brian S. Smith, Matthew Parker, Jesse Dillon, Jay Abramovitch, Steven Barker, Robby Burridge, Matt Zachary, Stacy Hurt, Greg Brown, Gary Puppa, Jason Manuge, Gary Bledsoe, Jeff Phillips, Erik Ingbretson, the late Jared McMillan, Laura Chavaree, Geoffrey Eich, Mark Elfers, Robert and Elaine Ramirez, Leah Robert, Sarah Nichols Kelley, Roger McCord, Brian Fitzgerald, Patty McCarthy, Martha Raymond, Jane Ashley, Lee Silverstein, Matt Dacey, Crystal Canney, Felicia Knight, Jenny Green, Trese Gloriod, Janelle Bretz, Suzi Pond, Erika Hanson Brown, Nancy Seybold, Manju George, the late Steve Schwarze, the late Todd Mercer, Julie Saliba Clauer, John Novack, Patti Sands, the Dempsey Center staff and board of directors, the late Kate Bergeron, Jodi Nofsinger, Elaine Gammon, Craig Bramley, the Berman & Simmons team, Dr. Evans, Dr. Pelletier, Dr. Mayo, Dr. Rutstein, Dr. Cusack, Dr. Clark, Dr. Le, Dr. Yurgelun, and Dr. Collins.

Sarah, the love for others that I give through Man Up to Cancer is only possible because of your love for me. I love you, now and always.

ABOUT THE AUTHOR

TREVOR MAXWELL

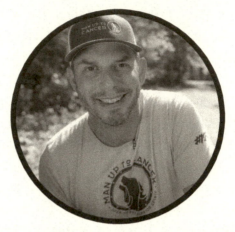

Trevor Maxwell was diagnosed with stage IV colon cancer in 2018, at age 41. He has undergone several major surgeries, chemotherapy, immunotherapy, and a clinical trial. Trevor has a background in newspaper journalism, communications, and public relations.

In January of 2020, Trevor founded Man Up to Cancer as a purpose-driven company and support community that inspires men to avoid isolation during the cancer journey.

He lives in Maine with his wife and two teenage daughters.

www.manuptocancer.com
www.instagram.com/cancerwolves
www.linkedin.com/in/manuptocancer
www.facebook.com/cancerwolves

Made in USA - North Chelmsford, MA
1344666_9798987178003
12.06.2022 1541